AN EXTRAORDINARY JOURNEY:

WHAT MATTERS AT THE END OF LIFE

AN EXTRAORDINARY JOURNEY:

WHAT MATTERS AT THE END OF LIFE

1ST EDITION

Teik Oh

MBBS, MD (Qld), FRACP, FANZCA, FCICM, FRCP, FRCPE, FRCA, FCARCSI, FCA SA
Emeritus Professor of Anaesthesia,
The University of Western Australia

ELSEVIER

ELSEVIER

Elsevier Australia. ACN 001 002 357
(a division of Reed International Books Australia Pty Ltd)
Tower 1, 475 Victoria Avenue, Chatswood, NSW 2067

ISBN: 978-0-7295-4374-3

National Library of Australia Cataloguing-in-Publication Data

A catalogue record for this book is available from the National Library of Australia

Senior Content Strategist: Larissa Norrie
Content Project Manager: Shivani Pal
Edited by Chris Wyard
Proofread by Tim Learner
Cover by Georgette Hall
Index by Innodata Indexing
Typeset by Toppan Best-set Premedia Limited
Printed in Australia

Last digit is the print number: 9 8 7 6 5 4 3 2 1

Contents

Foreword

The role of intensive care clinicians in treating critically ill patients has changed significantly over the evolution of this relatively young medical specialty.

Originally charged with providing mechanical ventilation for patients with acute respiratory failure caused by polio, clinical priorities evolved to provide expert resuscitation and vital organ support for patients with life-threatening organ failure. The establishment of dedicated educational and training programs in parallel with advanced technology resulted in the expansion and scope of intensive care units (ICUs) with reductions in mortality caused by previously lethal medical conditions.

However, increasing clinical demand and changing patient demographics has resulted in increasing numbers of terminally ill patients being admitted to and treated in the ICU – as a consequence of underlying acute illness or primarily as part of the dying process. As a result, there is an increasing expectation and requirement that intensive care clinicians engage in effective, compassionate and patient-centred end-of-life care.

A comprehensive textbook on the scale and scope of end-of-life care in the ICU is timely. Drawing on a lifetime of dedication to intensive care medicine, Teik Oh's name has become synonymous with his craft, not least through the publication of his seminal textbook – *Oh's Intensive Care Manual* – that informed and inspired generations of intensive care clinicians worldwide.

Teik's reflections on '*an extraordinary journey*' focusing on end-of-life care in the intensive care unit provide a comprehensive, yet exquisite, overview of what has become one of the most challenging, yet clinically important, aspects of modern intensive care practice.

Covering the broad range of clinical, ethical, societal and legal imperatives of end-of-life care, this book will become a key companion to the *manual,* but also as a stand-alone tome to facilitate and educate any clinician involved in a fundamental human right – the right to receive the best care at the end of life – when this occurs in an unfamiliar environment such as the intensive care unit.

John Myburgh AO
MBBCh, DSc, PhD, FCICM, FAHMS, FAICD
Professor of Intensive Care Medicine,
University of New South Wales

Preface

This book has its genesis in the legalisation of euthanasia, a common topic in Australia from 2017 to 2019. Proponents and opponents offered their strong views in gatherings, forums and all forms of media. Both sides pushed some arguments that contained incorrect facts and misinformation which muddied the debate and spread unease and confusion. I decided to write an article on euthanasia to explain the issues factually, without taking sides. In doing so, I realised that many issues in healthcare affect euthanasia, and at that point decided to write a book on matters that are important at the end of life, the last *extraordinary journey* we all must make.

In end-of-life care, families want to extend their loved one's life, but they struggle with defining what is acceptable 'humane' care and unacceptable 'heroic' care that precludes a 'good death'. Their medical goals may differ from those of the doctors, who sometimes do not know how to ascertain what they want. The families will face challenges and ask myriad questions such as:

How can they be sure of his prognosis?
How did they make this decision?
What about his living will?
How can he be brain dead!?
Can they withdraw treatment?
What are our rights?
Shouldn't they seek our consent first?
Can we request euthanasia?
What are our choices?
Why can't the hospital allow our choice?

This book addresses these questions and issues in language we all can understand. It describes the decisions doctors make based on principles of medical reasoning, ethics, consent and legal precedence as presented.

I drew upon case histories in my clinical experience to elucidate scenarios such as consent, autonomy, withholding or withdrawing treatment, 'living wills' and distributive justice. The clinical scenarios also explain frequently misunderstood topics such as brain death, vegetative states and deaths wrongly labelled as euthanasia.

I wrote this book for both healthcare professionals and lay readers to comprehend the *extraordinary journey*. As a specialist in Intensive Care Medicine and Anaesthesia, I know about patients' and families' experiences of critical illness in the ICU, where many *extraordinary journeys* are made. My aim was to help patients, families and carers understand end-of-life in hospitals; what matters to us, what choices we face and how decisions are made. If we understand each other's perspectives better, families can better navigate the alien hospital environment, and their loved ones' *extraordinary journey* may be more likely to be spiritual, dignified and good.

I wish to thank my wife Dide, my children Kazia and Stefan and their families for their support, John Rowe for his advice and help, John Myburgh for his Foreword and Larissa Norrie and Shivani Pal at Elsevier in producing the book.

Emeritus Professor Teik Oh AM
Perth, Western Australia, May 2020.

Introduction

When we think of death, we imagine ourselves sur-
rounded by loving friends, the room filled with quietude
that comes from nothing more to say; all business
finished; our eyes shining with love and with a whisper
of profound wisdom as to the transiency of life, we
settle back into the pillow, the last breath escaping
with a vast 'Ahh!' as we depart gently into the night.[1]

Walter Levine (1937–), US entrepreneur diagnosed
in 1991 with multiple myeloma and bladder cancers,
who after a stem cell transplant continues
to be in full remission (2017).

*

If an art gallery were to host an exhibition on 'Life', it would
display its paintings on death and dying, called 'Life's last journey'
in the final room of the gallery tour, appropriately next to the
exit and the souvenir shop. Some pictures would depict the last
stage of life, the *end-of-life* period, or, as called by some, the
twilight zone or *grey zone*. Many paintings would show a peaceful
death at home surrounded by family, what we would consider a
'good death'. Others might show death associated with suffering,
such as in Pieter Brueghel the Elder's *The triumph of death*,
Caravaggio's *Judith beheading Holofernes*, Andy Warhol's *Big electric
chair* and Goya's gruesome *Saturn devouring his son* – all 'bad
deaths'. That exhibition would make us think that deaths, just
like lives, might be good or bad. We may have been taught to
avoid talking about death, a taboo subject to be viewed with
dread, distaste and dismay. Instead of the words 'death' and 'dying',

1

we use euphemisms like 'expire', 'pass away' and 'terminal illness'. We fear pain and the isolation, loneliness and bleakness that dying brings – a bad death. Above all, what we fear most is the fear of the unknown. But death is part of life, indeed the main event. If death is inevitable with no escape, why should we ignore the elephant in our living room? Should we instead reflect on how we would like to die? Why not consider what matters affect the course of our dying process? How can we make our *extra-ordinary journey* from the known to the unknown less fearful and more accepting, perhaps even serene – a good death?

What we know today is that most deaths in developed countries occur in hospitals. In the 19th century, nearly all deaths transpired at home, but the numbers gradually changed. By the 1950s, only half of all deaths occurred at home, falling further to less than a quarter by the start of this 21st century. This proportion is even lower in Australia, where of the 160,000 deaths each year only 14% die at home, a third die in residential care facilities and over half of us die in hospitals.[2] The reasons most of us now die in hospitals are complex but centre around health services, social changes and disease trajectories. Our health system is consequently modelled on illness events that require treatment in hospitals, with the greatest health costs skewed towards the last months of life, culminating in end-of-life care. We can make choices through wills and powers of attorney on matters *after* our death (such as funerals, burials and bequeathals), but there are limits to our choices in hospital end-of-life care, even despite our preferences in advance care directives. Thus we are unlikely to die a 'good death' at home – as envisioned by Walter Levine – surrounded by family in our quiet bedroom and at peace with the world. We should then think about what matters influence our dying in hospitals.

Observational studies of end-of-life care today suggest variances in the care of patients dying in the hospital setting.[3] The care of these patients is not always optimal or of sufficient quality to reliably address their needs or expectations. These reports in general are from the hospice literature. End-of-life care in acute care hospital settings, with their complex and fragmented service delivery, medicalisation of death and lack of training, may even be worse.[4] Apart from treatment and hospital processes, hospital staff and patients may not consider other broad issues that impact on dying. In this context of deficiencies in our healthcare system, euthanasia may then appear to some as a 'better alternative' when death beckons. As the numbers of people dying in Australian hospitals are likely to exponentially increase over the next decades, there is a need to improve hospital end-of-life care,[5] and it helps to know what matters.

This book offers a compilation of reflections on death and dying in hospitals. The *Collins English dictionary* defines 'reflections' as *thoughts, considerations, comments, or writings about a particular subject*. Reflections in this book address matters in end-of-life care in hospital and the choices that patients, families and health professionals face in that extraordinary journey, and are grouped into six themes.

Part I covers the 'Twilight Zone' with three chapters. *Chapter 1 End of life* describes the decision making and choices that doctors, patients and families face in that period. *Chapter 2 Ethics in death and dying* defines death and explains the ethical principles including autonomy (the principle of self-determination), and *Chapter 3 Advance care directives* explains the legal and practical issues of one's premorbid preferences for care.

Part II covers 'Futility' with *Chapter 4* explaining *do not resuscitate* orders and *Chapter 5 Prognostications* explaining outcome predictions. *Chapter 6 Withdrawing treatment* describes the ethical and legal arguments for this contentious and distressing choice.

Part III covers the theme 'Communication' with *Chapter 7 Communication* explaining how good communication underpins quality medical care. *Chapter 8 Informed consent* describes this mandatory and integral component of patient-centred care.

Part IV covers 'Death' in three chapters. *Chapter 9 Brain death and vegetative states* explains the causes, diagnoses and differences between these conditions that confuse many people. *Chapter 10 Euthanasia* presents arguments for and against the mother-of-all medical controversies today and *Chapter 11 Organ donation* explains the process of gifting life-saving organs that can, in return, give meaning to the death of the deceased and comfort to the family.

Part V 'Faiths' covers religion in *Chapter 12 Religions at the end of life* and cultures in *Chapter 13 Cultures and ethnicities*. Death is not metaphysical but rather deeply personal; religious or cultural views of families may not accord with contemporary hospital medicine.

Part VI 'Health Services' is the final theme, with four chapters. Away from home as hospital patients, our health system and decisions made by the hospital staff shape our dying. Rules, bureaucracy and institutional cultures drive our health system, our hospitals and our end-of-life care. *Chapter 14 The healthcare system* and *Chapter 15 The intensive care unit* describe that maze of a system. *Chapter 16 Distributive justice* explains how valuable resources are allocated to deliver our care. Finally, and unfortunately, deaths in hospitals can occur because of errors, as described in *Chapter 17 Medical mishaps*.

As most deaths in Australia occur in hospitals, the book's principal setting is the intensive care unit (ICU), the scene of many end-of-life events. The reflections also contain stories of patients to illustrate issues being discussed. They are based on true case histories (although, in some, times and locations have been changed) though the characters' names and characteristics are fictional. Each chapter is self-contained and chapters can be read in any order, but some issues may overlap.

Some writers criticise doctors for the poor way some patients die: doctors who over-treat 'aggressively', miscommunicate options of care and pay scant attention to the wishes of patients and families. This book does not join that chorus. A good death is 'to die for' and can be difficult to coordinate in our segmented health system but, with few exceptions, doctors and nurses want that for their patients as much as for themselves. They are players in the game of life too, and they are in the same team.

I wrote this book for the health professionals and those under their care – patients and their families. My aim was to help all of us understand more about dying and the end of life in hospitals: what matters to us, what choices we face and how decisions are made. If the traveller, the family and the carers have a clearer view of the landscape to understand each other's perspectives better, *the extraordinary journey* may be more likely to be spiritual, dignified and good.

References

1. Walter T. *The revival of death*. Abingdon, UK: Routledge; 1994. p. 80.
2. Swerissen H, Duckett S. *Dying well*. Carlton, VIC: Grattan Institute; 2014.

3. Clark K, Collier A, Currow DC. Dying in Australian hospitals: will a separate national clinical standard improve the delivery of quality care? *Aust Health Rev* 2014;39:202.

4. The SUPPORT Principal Investigators. A controlled trial to improve care for seriously ill hospitalized patients. The study to understand prognoses and preferences for outcomes and risks of treatments (SUPPORT). *JAMA* 1995;274:1591.

5. Commission on Safety and Quality in Health Care. *National Consensus Statement: essential elements for safe and high-quality end-of-life care.* Sydney, NSW: ACSQHC; 2015.

Twilight Zone

CHAPTER 1

End of life

When the fat lady stops singing

I'm not afraid of death; I just don't want to be there when it happens.[1]

Woody Allen (1935–), American director, writer,
actor, comedian and musician

*

In medicine, *end of life* is known as the time period before death up to the death itself of a patient with an irreversible terminal illness or condition that has become advanced, progressive and incurable. This terminal phase of existence is sometimes called the *twilight zone* or the *grey zone* – the threshold between life and death.

*

'In the end they stopped everything. Pulled out all tubes and she passed.'

Mike Cook, my neighbour, was recounting how his grandmother had died in an interstate hospital, two days after a stroke. We had been talking about the death of Pope John Paul II on 2 April 2005.

'Like the Pope; peaceful really, in her sleep, all of us there. That's how I want to go when the fat lady stops singing.' Mike cocked an eyebrow. 'The doctors kept mentioning "*end-of-life care*". You're an ICU doctor, Tom. Is this what end of life is about? What is end-of-life care anyway? Can we choose how to die? Do you doctors ordain death? Do you doctors choose how to die yourselves?', he asked, looking pleased with such a clever question.

*

We stood at bed 9 on the Monday morning ward round, surrounding a thin, bald, middle-aged man lying in bed. An oral tracheal tube poked out of his mouth, connected to a bedside ventilator by twin corrugated hoses. His chest rose and fell rhythmically with each respiratory cycle. A large monitor sat on a shelf above his head, showing his vital signs: four green lines dancing across the dark screen competing for attention with evanescent numbers on the left margin. Various tubes – infusing fluids or monitoring blood pressures – invaded his arms, and a urine bag hung on a bed rail. A long bench demarcated one side of the bed area, with charts, kidney dishes, syringes, fluid bottles and dressings crowding its shelves. The man appeared asleep, but he opened his eyes when he heard us. I nodded to him and gave him a smile, and we moved away out of earshot. Dr Josh Shaw, who was on duty over the weekend, presented this new admission to Dr Milton Franks, Dr Paul Constable, Dr Rachel Lim and Rosemary Smith, the charge nurse. Milton was our respected senior consultant and Paul was our new consultant. Josh and Rachel were our registrars – trainees in intensive care medicine.

'Jim Hockaday, 62 years old. Admitted yesterday noon. Motor neuron disease, ALS, diagnosed three years ago. He was a patient here six months ago', Josh said.

Motor neuron disease is a progressive, terminal neurological condition. The most common form, amyotrophic lateral sclerosis (ALS), features degeneration and death of neurons in the brain and spinal cord. Transmission of messages from the brain to control movements of voluntary muscles decreases. The muscles gradually weaken and atrophy, and afflicted patients progressively lose their strength and ability to move their limbs. They eventually become unable to breathe effectively when their chest and diaphragm muscles fail. It afflicts two to three victims in every 100,000 people between 40 and 60 years of age. Patients have no impairment of mind or intelligence, or functioning of their eyes, bladder and bowel. Most die from respiratory failure, within three to five years from the onset of symptoms. The cause of this devastating disease is unknown and there is no effective cure.

'Yes, I remember him', Milton said. 'He came in with a chest infection. We didn't have to ventilate him though.'

'This time it's worse: another chest infection. His PO_2 was in the low 50s with PCO_2 in the 60s. I discussed with Tom', Josh said, nodding to me, 'and I intubated him'.

'His hypoxia and carbon dioxide retention were that severe, he was about to cardiac arrest', I said, a bit defensively, to explain why we initiated mechanical ventilation.

'Do we know what he and his family want?', Paul asked.

'We didn't know in ED; still don't', I said. 'Ambos brought him in without his wife. She came in later and said that he had made no advance care directives.' Josh Shaw provided more clinical details and we moved to the next bed.

I had decided to resuscitate Jim Hockaday without knowing his wishes for managing his crippling condition. He might, with antibiotics, recover but we would struggle to wean him off the ventilator, as the weaning success rate with ALS is less than 50%. That he had not required assisted ventilation in his previous admission swayed my decision. In a life-threatening emergency, doctors should provide life-saving interventions if the patient's preferences are unknown.[2] Once the person's condition is stabilised, their preferences or those of their substitute decision maker (SDM), if known, should apply. Without ventilation, Jim Hockaday would have died within a few hours.

Despite our previous advice to him, Jim had made no written advance care directive. His wife Betty informed me that, as his breathing efforts deteriorated over the past six months, he had expressed to her his wish for mechanical ventilation if needed. His demeanour during physiotherapy certainly suggested this, showing eagerness to please in his breathing exercises. Over the next four days his chest infection improved, and we started the weaning process. He exhausted himself in trying to breathe but, just as we feared, made no progress and soon developed another chest infection. After three weeks of weaning attempts, he remained incapable of effective spontaneous breathing. His chest infection worsened. He stopped cooperating with the physiotherapists, and became restless, fidgeting in bed. His eyes looked dull and blank, registering no interest in what was happening around him. With further deterioration of his condition, his mental state became clouded. Dr Will Mullins, head of respiratory medicine, and Dr Tim Mason, consultant neurologist, who had been following his progress, agreed with the futility of continuing ventilator support. Jim Hockaday had entered the twilight zone.

*

End of life

How long is 'end of life'? There is no definitive length of time that encapsulates end of life, as diseases and injuries have unpredictable progressions and exacerbations. In hospices and palliative care wards, it may be a few weeks or months, and, in general hospital wards, days or even hours in the ICU. The Australian Commission on Safety and Quality in Health Care (ACSQHC) defines this period as 12 months (including periods of exacerbated illness that may recover), but incorporates a short-term component of days and weeks, when clinical deterioration is irreversible.[3] Obviously, in an acute hospital, end-of-life care concerns the latter group. Jim Hockaday's end of life would be the last days of his life, after three weeks of intensive care that proved futile in restoring spontaneous breathing.

Today, short-term end-of-life care is practised mostly in hospitals. End-of-life practices historically evolved as palliative care within hospices dedicated to the dying process, and were adapted as end-of-life care to nursing homes, hospitals and even private homes. However, introducing and delivering palliative care to these settings are not without challenges; patients, families and staff sometimes experience a poor dying transition without the benefits of a good death.

The majority (over half) of the 160,000 Australians who die each year die in hospitals,[4] with deaths representing less than 1% of all admissions into hospitals. Deaths in the ICU account for 13% of all deaths in the hospital, although less than 2% of hospital inpatients are admitted to ICU during their hospital stay. Hence end-of-life considerations are important aspects of ICU care, especially when many patients cannot communicate their wishes. End-of-life care in the ICU setting often follows withdrawal of treatment when it is deemed futile: a U-turn trajectory of care and a 'cure-to-comfort' transition. Death may be swift, but is often complicated by an unpredictable short dying phase. This short timeframe within a dynamic clinical environment in the ICU poses difficulties for staff to prepare the patient and their families for a quality death. The setting imposes emotional and physical stresses on the families, which can be worsened by inconsistencies in decision making to withdraw, withhold or alter treatment and when to do so.

Dying in hospital differs from dying at home or in nursing homes. Many factors in the healthcare systems of hospitals (see Chapter 14 The healthcare system), such as administrative structures, costs, financing, bureaucracy and policies, determine bedside care. These factors may pose potential adverse consequences for patients and their families. Hospitals can also manipulate the time of death in end of life, by decisions on whether and when to continue or stop treatment, and on what grounds, as exemplified by ICU practices.

Is *end-of-life care* the same as *palliative care*? These two terms can be confusing, but they are different concepts. End-of-life care focuses on helping a patient nearing death to live this last period of life as well as possible, with an aim of allowing them to die as comfortably as possible and with dignity. Palliative care is multidisciplinary, specialised medical care for a patient with any serious illness. It focuses on providing relief from distressing symptoms, with psychological, social and spiritual support for the patient and family. This is a holistic approach, treating the patient as a 'whole' person. Palliative care may be indicated early in the illness, which need not be life threatening and is not limited to, or reserved for, the end-of-life period. End-of-life care comes bundled with palliative care.

*

The interview room was a quiet room fitted out with standard hospital furnishings: steel waiting room chairs with plastic seats, two wooden coffee tables and a water dispenser standing in a corner. Boxes of paper tissues lay on the tables with piles of old magazines donated by the staff. Reserved for family conversations, the room was used to explain medical issues, communicate good and bad news and seek informed consent. The nurses called it the 'crying room' because the walls witnessed much grieving. Two of Elizabeth Durack's paintings hung on one wall. Donated by a grateful patient, the prints portrayed indigenous figures in the harsh, arid, beautiful landscape of Western Australia's Kimberley region. They provided a much-needed spiritual serenity to balance the clinical, sombre hospital ambience.

Betty Hockaday was a slim and elegant middle-aged woman. They met when she was a dental nurse in Jim's practice, and they worked as a team throughout their 35-year marriage. There were no children. In the past week, she had realised her husband's bleak prognosis. Her shoulders sagged more each day as she became increasingly dispirited. The demands of coping with his suffering, and the physical toll from poor sleep and travelling multiple times each day to the hospital, had added dark rings under her eyes.

I guided her by her elbow to a seat. Touch is an important undertaking for a doctor. A handshake commonly provides the first connection with the patient or relative. Apart from the physical examination, a handshake or light touch on their arm or shoulder, particularly in the presence of emotional distress, can suggest to them that their doctor is aware of their distress and is present to be supportive.

'Betty, we spoke the last three days about Jim's condition getting worse. You can see that now', I said. 'His infection is spreading and his lungs and kidneys are now starting to fail. He's become restless, and we had to increase his sedation. You can see that he's hard to rouse now. All of us here, and the chest physician and neurologist, agree that Jim can never again breathe on his own. If we continue, it will only briefly prolong his life. It's only a matter of time before he gets overwhelmed with infections.' I paused. 'I think Jim has had enough. I can't check with him because he is not mentally alert. What would Jim want *now*, you think?'

She looked at me in silence, and then turned her gaze to the floor. Her eyes misted, but she held back her tears. She kept stroking her wedding ring. I didn't say anything more.

'I don't know what to say … to do. I … I only want him to live', she said softly. 'Is there no hope? Won't dialysis buy some time? Will a palliative care specialist help?' Her eyes looked up, pleading.

'I am so sorry Betty. Dialysis won't even save his kidneys, and Jim is receiving palliative care. With his progressive multiple organ failure, we can keep him alive for a few days at the most, but that would not be in his best interests', I replied. I did not mention that we could legally withdraw futile treatment if judged in the patient's best interests.

'Are you saying that you want to stop the ventilator?' She looked at her wedding ring, deep in her thoughts, and then looked up and slowly nodded. 'Stop the ventilator. Please don't let him suffer. *Please let him die a good death.*'

Betty contacted Jim's three brothers. We arranged for our social workers and the Hockadays' local Anglican priest to provide social and spiritual support to her. Much paperwork had been completed two days ago in anticipation of his death. The time was set for early that evening. Rosemary Smith moved him into a single room and Jacinta, the bed nurse, drew the curtains. We switched off all monitoring devices, and removed leads and vascular lines except for a morphine drip. The brothers arrived and gathered at the bedside. Jacinta explained to the family what was happening at each step. Jim Hockaday by then was comatose. Milton, Rachel and I occasionally showed our presence in the room. At 7.00 pm, Milton disconnected the ventilator. Jim Hockaday started breathing on his own: rapid, shallow, weak, barely discernable breaths. He did not cough. Betty hugged him and his brothers held his hands as his skin discoloration deepened. Jim stopped breathing after two or three minutes, and his heart stopped six minutes later. He never regained consciousness and died surrounded by his family.

*

A good death

Betty Hockaday expressed her wish for a 'good death' for her husband. A 'good death' or 'dying well' is indeed what all of us would wish for ourselves when we travel our last journey. Multiple determinants – including patient and family perceptions, autonomy, setting and end-of-life care delivered – can influence a 'good death'. But what is 'a good death'? The media has said much about good end-of-life care, with a wide usage of rhetorical terms like 'ending suffering', 'dying with dignity', 'quality of life', 'dying well' and a 'good death', but the definitions of these terms are imprecise and unclear. Patients near death and their families can have vague ideas that their impending death can somehow be 'good' and 'natural', which they mean to be peaceful, pain free and easy. And yet they often perceive death to be fearful, difficult, painful and demeaning. At the end of life, as the patient's condition deteriorates, there is often uncertainty about what to do, and ambiguity about what the medical goals are, on the side of both the family *and* the doctors. Understanding what the patient and family want becomes significantly important.

What does the patient want?

The views of patients and families for end-of-life care to achieve 'a good death' are summarised in seven main patient-centred themes (*see Box*).[5,6]

Patient-centred Views of Dying Well

- Autonomy to be involved in, and control over, decisions about their care.
- Access to high-quality care by skilled staff.
- Access to the right services when needed.
- Support for physical, emotional, social and spiritual needs.
- The right people to know their wishes at the right time.
- Support for the people important to them.
- To be cared for and die in the place of their choice.

The most important wish is that of autonomy, the right to decide about one's own care. Patient autonomy is a cornerstone of medical practice today. The principle originated from the Nuremberg Code in August 1947,[7] which was the Nuremberg Tribunal's response to Nazi atrocities in medical research. The Code, which focused on the conduct of medical research and the rights of sick patients and healthy subjects to engage in medical research, gave rise to patients' rights. Over the next two decades, patients' rights and patients' self-determination became key issues in healthcare. The US Federal Patient Self-Determination Act in 1990 mandated that all hospital patients must be informed of their right to make treatment choices, and this patients' right was similarly enacted as laws of rights and consent by other developed countries.

*

What do families want?

Conflict sometimes transpires between treatment preferred by the incapacitated patient and those of doctor-dominated decisions. Awkward situations arise when the family cannot agree or decide on treatment preferences asked by the doctors. Most families do not understand how hospitals work, and can be overwhelmed by the seemingly endless available interventions that they face, although faith in medical treatment is usually strong. Families know *what they want,* just like Betty Hockaday – their loved one to not die or to not suffer – but they do not know *what to want* when facing care choices. Some may even feel distressed by the burden exerted on them to make decisions, with a perception that they are asked to take responsibility for ending life, rather than exercising their option for end-of-life care. Others make choices that cannot be implemented (see later is this chapter). Families' culture, religion and socioeconomic status to a large extent determine their choices. All are torn between wanting to extend their loved one's life with effective interventions and not wanting excessive technological interventions to preclude a 'good death'. They struggle with defining acceptable 'humane' care and unacceptable 'heroic' care. How can John and Jane determine, for example, whether mechanical ventilation, an infusion of heart stimulants, dialysis or nasogastric feeding is a 'natural' standard of care for their dying mother and, if so, under what conditions? Or are these 'aggressive' interventions that artificially prolong life and delay death? At what point does a 'natural' treatment become 'burdensome'? Even the terms 'life support treatment' and 'life-sustaining treatment' are not always easy to explain or understand. A 'life support' or 'life-sustaining' treatment is not a single discrete activity or procedure, and has no defining boundaries. Also, when families themselves do not know their preferences, doctors sometimes do not know how to scrutinise what they want.

*

'It's been a bad week. Firstly Millie Coogan, then John Wellesley and today, Jim Hockaday. We ought to open a funeral parlour service', Rosemary Smith said, shaking her head with a grimace. 'Two of the staff are really feeling washed out. I've asked Jessica Prior for help.'

Rosemary was referring to the deaths we had that week: three end-of-life events with three withdrawals of treatment. Jim Hockaday's motor disease was an uncommon cause of death, whereas Millie Coogan died from the most common cause of death in ICUs: overwhelming sepsis. She was a 70-year-old with a history of diverticular disease (diverticula or small pouch defects in her colon). She had presented to the emergency department two weeks previously with bowel perforation – a complication of diverticulitis or infection of the abnormal pouches – and underwent emergency surgery. Postoperatively, sepsis from her presenting abdominal soiling worsened despite antibiotics and became blood-borne, and she developed multiorgan failure.

John Wellesley was an 85-year-old retiree who collapsed from a cardiac arrest in a large shopping centre. A passer-by had rendered immediate cardiopulmonary resuscitation, aided soon after by paramedics stationed within the mall itself. He was brought to the hospital emergency department unconscious and intubated, where a diagnosis of acute myocardial infarction was confirmed. The overall survival rate of cardiac arrests outside hospitals is poor, at less than 8%. This was evident in John Wellesley in the ICU where his hypoxic brain injury from cardiac arrest – despite prompt and excellent resuscitation – progressed to brain death in the next 36 hours. All treatment ceased when brain death was confirmed.

*

Making hard decisions

In the past week, the ICU staff had experienced three end-of-life events with the patients' families. John Wellesley's family had no treatment options. He was brain dead, and thus legally dead (Chapter 9 Brain death and vegetative states). We stopped all treatment and would have done so regardless of what his family might have requested. Millie Coogan's family and Betty Hockaday had only one choice: to continue or to withdraw futile treatment when death was imminent. They did not request ongoing treatment, and we did not offer this, but it was up to us to inform and explain why that would have been futile. We made decisions in the patients' best interests, and their families agreed with us. I believe that Jim Hockaday, Millie Coogan and John Wellesley would have too.

Decision making in reality is often not deliberate or premeditated, and at times may have no practical bearing on end-of-life care. Emergencies and pragmatism often determine decisions in the best interests of the patient. Doctors may make decisions with or without family discussions, but the days of paternalism – where the doctor is the sole decision maker – are no more. Families never want to choose death, but many accept death, usually after discussions with their doctors when they realise that death is inevitable.

End-of-life experiences are stressful for both families and staff. There are reports of burnout and posttraumatic stress disorder (PTSD) experienced by ICU doctors and nurses.[8,9] Doctors are challenged to compartmentalise their professional thinking from their personal feelings when making difficult decisions in end-of-life care. They, with nurses and other health professionals, experience feelings of frustration, sadness and grief at different stages of end-of-life care. Rosemary Smith had requested Jessica Prior, a psychotherapist, to provide counselling to our staff. She was a tremendous asset in counselling ICU patients, their families and, also importantly, our staff in times of severe stress.

*

Limits of patient autonomy

Patients and families at times question whether doctors always follow their choices. The answer is no. Although the *principle* of patient autonomy is absolute in modern medicine, there are limits in *application*. Individual doctors' decisions, the health system and hospital culture, with their myriad regulations, bureaucracy and professional standards, can limit patient autonomy to a narrower scope of medical choices. Ethics and laws are added constraints. For example, at the heart of a hospital-centred healthcare system, a patient choice to die at home is impractical and unrealistic, or to die from assisted suicide is illegal (Chapter 10 Euthanasia). It is arguable whether true, complete, free patient autonomy can ever be delivered in today's end-of-life care. Unsurprisingly, sociologists and health commentators have criticised how hospitals manage dying, the procedures for dying and the healthcare bureaucracy in which dying takes place. Some have expressed the desirability of patients to choose their hospitals to be admitted when sick, and to choose doctors to treat them when dying. For seriously ill patients, these choices are unrealistic in public health systems, as explained in Chapter 14 The healthcare system, but the critics may have a point about deficiencies in quality end-of-life care. Indeed, the difficulties surrounding end-of-life care may be 'incurable' in major hospitals. In the 1990s, five US hospitals conducted an end-of-life care study in two stages over four years – the SUPPORT study.[10] The first stage recorded deficiencies in communication, pain control, knowing patients' preferences for resuscitation, length of stay in ICU and excessive use of aggressive treatment and mechanical ventilation. The hospitals then implemented improvement strategies to address the shortcomings via multiple contacts between staff and patients and their families. The second-stage study showed, unexpectedly, that the positive interventions *failed* to improve care, patient outcomes or characteristics of death. Also, it showed that advance care directives had no significant effect on limiting resuscitation efforts at time of death. This gives rise to an interesting and sobering *non sequitur* view that *full-scale* patient autonomy may not be attainable or even appropriate in end-of-life care.

End-of-life care

Mike had asked, 'What is end-of-life care anyway?' Many countries like Australia have guidelines in providing end-of-life care to help caregivers and families.[11] Particularly helpful are the roles and behaviours of doctors and nurses. Doctors sometimes participate less than they should once the decision to stop treatment is made, whereas nurses are often the true heroes. Few general hospitals have dedicated, specialist palliative care teams who can come in, engage and support. End-of-life care has three goals: to provide palliative care for individual dying patients and their families to minimise suffering and distress, to develop healthcare system-wide strategies to ensure best practice in palliative care wherever a patient is dying; and to support the healthcare staff who care for dying patients. We all need to think and talk about the dying process, the dying person and ways to manage treatment, prepare for death and, ultimately, embrace death.

End-of-life guidelines recommend that we recognise and identify end-of-life patients so that dying patients, their families and their healthcare staff can reorientate their priorities and achieve their goals in order to provide appropriate end-of-life care. In many clinical situations in the ICU, imminent death can be predicted – for example, in a patient with rapidly deteriorating failure of organs. Indices and guides to prognosticate the risk of death are available (Chapter 5 Prognostications) to help identify end-of-life care patients, although they are not useful as sole predictors.

End-of-life care must cater for both patient and family. Best practice focuses on supporting them both, and does not include the family merely as an afterthought. Care attends to the physical as well as the psychosocial and spiritual concerns of patients and their families, and the care extends into the bereavement period. Help from counsellors like Jessica Prior is invaluable. Good teamwork between healthcare professionals is essential, and good communication with families is vital. The latter requires engagement in timely, consistent and compassionate conversations and in providing information (Chapter 7 Communication). Families struggle to understand medical information. Doctors have a wealth of medical knowledge, but they must understand that families have great difficulty in interpreting and understanding the *same* pieces of information. Also, in conveying treatment plans, doctors focus on the next potential move such as withdrawing treatment and preparing for death, whereas families look at the whole picture including the hope of survival and avoidance of suffering.

Palliative treatment plans such as in managing pain and physical problems, and in withdrawing treatment, must be addressed. Promoting the comfort of the dying person includes managing pain, agitation, shortness of breath, respiratory secretions, mouth and skin care, bladder and bowel care, and nausea and vomiting. Treatment is individualised. Interventions that are burdensome or do not improve the dying person's comfort should also be stopped if possible. All patients and families fear pain. Effective treatment is critical with morphine or related medications, although it may hasten death by causing respiratory depression in a spontaneously breathing patient. Pertinent to this is the *doctrine of double effect*: that if doing something morally good has a morally bad side effect, that good deed is justified provided that the bad side-effect was not intended (Chapter 2 Ethics in death and dying). Accordingly, giving morphine in this situation is ethically and legally acceptable. Excessive secretions – unfortunately called the 'death rattle' – can upset families and should be properly managed. In withdrawing ventilation, the ventilation volume and oxygen can be incrementally decreased, or the ventilator can be switched off, or the tracheal tube removed, depending on discussions with the family. There is no emotionally easy or 'best' way to disconnect from the ventilator.

The relief of suffering also includes the relief of psychological, social and spiritual distress. 'Spirituality' has its own meaning in each individual, but in general is a broad term relating to our thoughts and feelings about our own being. It is a sense of peace and purpose, based more on individual philosophies and developing beliefs around the meaning of life and connection with others. Spirituality is shaped more by culture than by established faiths.

Staff must also be aware of the religious and cultural sensitivities of the patients and their families (Chapter 12 Religions at the end of life, Chapter 13 Cultures and ethnicities). These beliefs are important in many individuals in the dying process, and to support their values is a component of quality end-of-life care especially in view of Australia's ethnic and cultural diversity. End-of-life experiences expose ICU staff to grief and suffering probably more than other workplaces, and they themselves must also be supported. Staff members normally draw on each other for their network of support. Staff debriefing sessions are recognised as important, but are not too common.

Advance care directives, if present, are important in making decisions on treatment choices (Chapter 3 Advance care directives). The ICU staff must be clear on when treatment has become futile and be able to communicate this to the family, and learn from them their wishes for the patient. Decisions to withdraw or withhold further treatment, or why an advance care directive cannot be implemented, must be clarified to the family. There is sometimes a fine dividing line between families feeling that their loved one had died after too much technological interventions and, on the other hand, that the doctors had been too quick to stop treatment with too little personal say on the family's part. In the US, less than 10% of the population have advance care directives, and in Australia this figure is 14%.[12] True, advance care directives may not resolve too many questions about how aggressive treatment at end of life should be. Many advance care directives do not explicitly state preferences for resuscitation such as a wish for a 'do not resuscitate' order. They are often too vague to be relevant or to give useful information about the patient's wishes. Some people also do not want their future treatment to be determined by previously written documents.

Old age and end-of-life practice

In Australia, patients aged 65 years or older make up over 40% of all hospital admissions, and this percentage is increasing each year.[13] Of hospital deaths, over 93% are patients aged 50 years or older and 55% are males. Hence old age is an end-of-life care issue in hospitals, and yet no one technically dies of old age.

*

The seminar room was a large room capable of seating 30 people, lecture-theatre style. It was where we were holding our weekly clinical review meeting, this time to review the deaths of Jim Hockaday, Millie Coogan and John Wellesley. Rachel Lim presented the cases at the lectern. Facing her were the ICU doctors, nurses and six medical students. Discussions about each patient had centred on what we could have done better in their end-of-life care, but no great ideas had been forthcoming.

'John Wellesley's autopsy showed a severe acute myocardial infarction – the official cause of death – secondary to coronary thrombosis', Rachel said. 'He had severe atherosclerosis, not surprising as he was a smoker, but he was 85! We had no choice but to admit him because he was already intubated when he arrived in ED. He was unconscious, breathing spontaneously, but his airway was compromised and he could not be extubated. He was 85 but, in essence, we were treating his heart disease. I checked the International Classification of Diseases (ICD),[14] which coordinates worldwide mortality and morbidity data used in many countries including Australia, and old age is not a disease. We can't sign a death certificate stating the cause of death as old age.

No one can officially die of old age. We all know that a continuum of conditions exists between ageing and disease, such as athero-sclerosis and osteoporosis. But we were officially treating a pathological condition – atherosclerosis – rather than old age. If age-related diseases are pathological conditions, can old age overall be one pathological condition? Should we treat aged patients aggressively because of their specific pathological conditions or should we refuse ICU admission routinely to let them die naturally of the single pathological condition of old age? Where is the dividing line? What is the correct end-of-life care?' She shrugged her shoulders with a bemused smile. Her points and questions flummoxed everyone into silence. It is difficult to categorise conditions found in elderly people, such as atherosclerosis, as normal or pathological. In practice, we consider old age with the presenting diagnosis and prognosis in deciding whether to admit to ICU and the level of treatment to administer in end-of-life care (see Chapter 16 Distributive justice).

*

Choosing a good death

We have to ask ourselves, how do we choose to die a 'good death'? For many of us, our last few months consume the greatest healthcare costs in our lifetime, but more effective alternatives of dying have not replaced our procedure-orientated, event-determined and hospital-centred model. We all fear dying in pain and dying alone. Consequently, autonomy and dignity are important for a 'good death', with our choices of where we die and who will be present, and supported by skilled management of our pain and discomfort. In reality, we usually cannot choose where to die, and coordinated and multidisciplinary end-of-life care can be difficult in our compartmentalised healthcare systems. This may explain how doctors choose to die. Dr Ken Murray, a retired family practice doctor, in an article in the *Wall Street Journal*,[15] wrote how most doctors choose to die at home with no 'heroic measures' and with less aggressive care than most people get at the end of their lives. A Stanford University study[16] disturbingly found that most doctors would choose a 'do not resuscitate' order for themselves when they are terminally ill, but some might pursue aggressive treatments for patients with the same prognosis while still believing that to be in their patients' best interests.

Australia is a less litigation-conscious society than the US and, in our practice, our doctors may be less likely to choose 'defensive' aggressive treatments for their patients in end-of-life care. Despite that, as a society, if we know more about dying and dying in our hospitals, our families would surely be more prepared for what to expect, and then how to respond, when each of us enters the twilight zone to make our last extraordinary journey.

*

Reflections

- End-of-life care has complex issues. Patient autonomy is paramount but is limited by many ethical, systemic and professional factors.
- When there are no advance care directives, families should communicate clearly their preferences in end-of-life care. In their considerations, the yardstick to use is: what is in the patient's best interests?
- Doctors' treatment decisions may not align with the patient's or family's preferences. They should explain to the family why a choice cannot be implemented. Their decisions are ultimately made using the same yardstick – in the patient's best interests. Withdrawal of futile treatment is legal if judged in the patient's best interests.
- End-of-life situations pose enormous stresses on family members and the healthcare staff.

References

1. Allen W. *Death: a comedy in one act*. New York: Samuel French; 1975.
2. Australian Health Ministers' Advisory Council. *Australian framework for advance care directives*. Rundle Mall, SA: AHMAC; 2011.
3. Commission on Safety and Quality in Health Care. *National consensus statement: essential elements for safe and high-quality end-of-life care*. Sydney, NSW: ACSQHC; 2015.
4. Australian Institute of Health and Welfare. *Deaths in Australian hospitals 2014–15*. Canberra, ACT: AIHW; 2017.

5. Australian Institute of Health and Welfare. *6.18 End-of-life care*. Australia's Health. Canberra, ACT: AIHW; 2016.
6. Victorian Government Department of Health. *Strengthening palliative care: policy and strategic directions 2011–2015*. Melbourne, VIC: DOH; 2012. http://docs2.health.vic.gov.au/docs/doc/26A45CD219CD1FA7CA2579B3007E54F5/$FILE/Strengthening%20palliative%20care%20implementation%20strategy.pdf.
7. Schuster E. Fifty years later: the significance of the Nuremberg Code. *N Engl J Med* 1997;337:1436.
8. Simpson N, Knott C. Stress and burnout in intensive care medicine: an Australian perspective. *Med J Aust* 2017;206:107–8.
9. Mealer M, Berg B, Rothbaum B, Moss M. Increased prevalence of post traumatic stress disorder symptoms in critical care nurses. *Am J Respir Crit Care Med* 2007;176(7):693–7.
10. The SUPPORT Principal Investigators. A controlled trial to improve care for seriously ill hospitalized patients. The study to understand prognoses and preferences for outcomes and risks of treatments (SUPPORT). *JAMA* 1995;274:159.
11. National EOL Framework Forum. *Health system reform and care at the end of life: a guidance document*. Canberra, ACT: Palliative Care Australia; 2010.
12. White B, Tilse C, Wilson J, Rosenman L, Strub T, Feeney R, et al. Prevalence and predictors of advance directives in Australia. *Intern Med J* 2014;44:975.
13. Australian Institute of Health and Welfare. *Admitted patient care 2014–15*. Australian Hospital Statistics. Canberra, ACT: AIHW; May 2017.
14. World Health Organization. *International Classification of Diseases ICD-11 (version: 04/2019)*. Geneva: WHO; 2019. https://icd.who.int/browse11/l-m/en.
15. Murray K. Why doctors die differently. *Wall Str J* 2012; February 25. http://online.wsj.com/article/SB10001424052970203918304577243321242833962.html.
16. Periyakoil VS, Neri E, Fong A, Kraemer H. Do unto others: doctors' personal end-of-life resuscitation preferences and their attitudes toward advance directives. *PLoS ONE* 2014;9(5):e98246.

2

Ethics in death and dying

Moralities in end of life

Death is not the greatest loss in life. The greatest loss is what dies inside us while we live.

Norman Cousins (1915–90), American journalist and author

*

The Australian Law Reform Commission in 1977 defined legal death as *circulatory death* or *brain death.* Death can also be categorised according to the manner causing death: *natural causes* as death of its own accord through age, terminal illness or disease; *accidental death* as death by misadventure that is unintended or unexpected; *homicide* as death of a person by premeditated murder; and *suicide* as death of a person intentionally acted upon by that person.

Definition of death

Man has struggled with defining death in history. In early societies until the 18th century, death was understood to be the separation of soul (or spirit) from the body. Timing of death was not specified; the physical signs preceded the liberation of the spirit from the body. Traditional death was then determined by the absence of the heartbeat and respiration – a biomedical determination – and a time of death could be documented. Death can then be considered an *event*. With advances in medicine such as cardiopulmonary resuscitation and mechanical ventilation, circulation and oxygenation could be restored in certain pulseless, non-breathing persons, thus returning a 'dead' person to life (albeit temporarily in some). Death is established only when irreversible, and death can then be considered a *condition*. While circulation and breathing have ceased, not all biological units (cells, tissues and organs) die simultaneously in synchrony. At the time of cardiorespiratory death of the person, the inherent basic processes of lower-level biological units continue for some time. Death can then be considered a *process*, although a time of death is certified.

The medical advances in the 1960s saw the survival of patients with irreversible coma and unresponsiveness who would previously have died. Organ transplantation was in its infancy, but the massive potential to save lives with donated organs was recognised. A definition of death was needed to limit treatment of persistent vegetative states and improve the opportunities for organ retrieval. The concept of 'brain death' was introduced by the Ad Hoc Committee of the Harvard Medical School[1] using the criteria of flat line reading on electroencephalogram (EEG) and a lack of blood circulation in the brain – the *Harvard criteria*. This definition of death by brain death was modified and has been accepted universally in the past 50 years (Chapter 9 Brain death and vegetative states).

Death is deeply personal. Each of us, with our families, deals with it according to our values and our communal customs; a one-size approach definitely does not fit all. According to Kübler-Ross,[a] we experience five emotional stages in dying: denial, anger, bargaining, depression and acceptance, but not necessarily all evoked, or in that order. These behaviours may be observed in patients in end-of-life care. When we are dying, we with our families can seek end-of-life care and palliative care, prepare our advance care directives and may even be able to plan how we

---

[a] Elisabeth Kübler-Ross (1926–2004) was a Swiss-American psychiatrist, a pioneer in near-death studies and the author of the ground-breaking book *On death and dying* (1969),[2] where she first discussed her theory of the five stages of grief.

die. However, death may come before our expected time, such as following an acute severe illness or a traumatic injury, and most of us will die in a hospital.

Medical advances have created ethical challenges for our doctors, our families and ourselves when we are dying. We are often confronted with difficult choices regarding treatment that may inadvertently prolong suffering and the dying process rather than result in recovery. Principles of medical ethics guide doctors in making morally acceptable treatment choices. Ethical principles are respected in our end-of-life care, but how we die may not be how we choose to die. Hence doctors need to be aware of potential ethical dilemmas and the strategies to avoid conflicts with patients and families.

*

Chronic obstructive pulmonary disease

'It's an old friend, Mr Jason Black', said Rachel Lim, her lips twisted in a wry expression. She was presenting in our ICU department's weekly clinical review meeting in the seminar room. She gave a summary of 70-year-old Jason Black's two previous admissions with respiratory failure over the past year. He had chronic obstructive pulmonary disease (COPD), a consequence of 52 years of heavy smoking. In his last admission six months previously, he required mechanical ventilation, but he almost died because we struggled to wean him off the ventilator. This time, he was admitted with another chest infection and respiratory failure. Wesley Thomas, the fourth member of our consultant team, had admitted him.

'Why did you take him?', Paul Constable asked.

'For a trial of care', Wesley said with a defensive ring in his voice, 'To try mask-ventilation, but not to intubate and ventilate.'

'I still would not have admitted him', Paul said. 'The last time, it took ages to wean him, and we were lucky, I reckon. I remember he was with us for 2 months and wreaked havoc with our bed shortage. I see that he has not given up smoking. Last time we asked him to make an advance care directive. Does he have one? It would make decision making easier.'

'No.' A debate followed, with the two registrars agreeing with Paul. Milton Franks and I were more circumspect.

*

COPD is a serious, progressive and disabling condition that limits air flow in the lungs. It includes emphysema (enlarged air sacs from tissue destruction) and chronic bronchitis (excessive mucus in airways), and smoking is the predominant cause. Half of all smokers will develop some form of air-flow limitation, and 15%–20% of smokers will develop severe lung problems. About 1 in 20 Australians aged 45 years and over have COPD, the fifth most common cause of death in 2017.[3] Around a billion dollars a year is spent in Australia treating COPD.[4] Men aged over 65 years who continue to smoke reduce their life expectancy by three and a half years; this is reduced further by almost six years in those with severe COPD similar to Jason Black's.[5] At 70 years, he had reached his predicted terminal period of life.

Recurrent admissions into ICU of smokers with COPD are always contentious issues. Ventilation of their damaged lungs is fraught with complications, and recovery can be unpredictable. Weaning off ventilation is long and arduous, often without success, and tying up a bed for weeks may block admitting new, 'more worthy' patients. Decision making to admit a COPD in respiratory failure should balance core ethical principles of *beneficence* and *distributive justice* – the fair allocation of medical resources, when full intensive care treatment can cost A$4000 to A$6000 per day. At times, a decision is made for a trial of assisted mask-ventilation only, as Wesley had made for Jason Black. How does one decide?

*

Medical ethics

Medical ethics are a set of moral principles, beliefs and values that guide us in making choices about medical care. At the core of medical ethics is our sense of right and wrong in caring for our patients. Ethical standards in medical care promote other important societal morals and values, such as social responsibility, compliance with the law, human rights and patients' rights, welfare and safety.

Medical ethics deal with norms in practising medicine. To help or improve the health of its people, the community grants doctors and healthcare professionals privileges that are not granted to the lay public. For example, doctors get to palpate and perform procedures on people's bodies; prescribe powerful, potentially lethal drugs; and decide how patient care is to be delivered, which patient should get which treatment, how much patients should be told about their condition, and who will die sooner and who will live a bit longer. These matters affect every human being at some point in each person's life. Without ethical guidelines or conduct, doctors may misuse or be careless with the power and privileges entrusted to them. Thus, considerations of medical ethics are among the most important and consequential in human life.

The Hippocratic Oath

Medical ethics today are based on two expositions: the *Hippocratic Oath* and *principlism*. Hippocrates (450–380 BCE), called 'the father of medicine' since antiquity, was a physician born about 2000 years ago who lived on the island of Cos in the Aegean Sea, then a centre of learning in ancient Greece. He is credited with a collection of medical writings, the *Corpus Hippocraticum*, which comprised descriptions of diseases, diagnoses, medical prescriptions, diets, health recommendations and his opinion on professional ethics – the Hippocratic Oath. This is one of the oldest binding documents in history, a code of conduct for doctors in which the medical profession has over centuries grounded the basics of professional practice. Some doctors today might consider the Hippocratic Oath to be immaterial in a contemporary medical world that has experienced huge scientific, political and social changes. Nonetheless, graduates of most medical schools still pledge this oath – some perhaps as a proforma ritual, redolent of tradition – and it still remains an oath of commitment to respect medical ethics in the practice of Western medicine. A modern version in common use that is more relevant to today's world was written by Louis Lasagna of Tufts University in 1964 (*see Box*).

The Hippocratic Oath (Lasagna 1964)[6]

I swear to fulfil, to the best of my ability and judgment, this covenant:

- I will respect the hard-won scientific gains of those physicians in whose steps I walk, and gladly share such knowledge as is mine with those who are to follow.
- I will apply, for the benefit of the sick, all measures [that] are required, avoiding those twin traps of overtreatment and therapeutic nihilism.
- I will remember that there is art to medicine as well as science, and that warmth, sympathy and understanding may outweigh the surgeon's knife or the chemist's drug.
- I will not be ashamed to say 'I know not', nor will I fail to call in my colleagues when the skills of another are needed for a patient's recovery.
- I will respect the privacy of my patients, for their problems are not disclosed to me that the world may know. Most especially must I tread with care in matters of life and death. If it is given me to save a life, all thanks. But it may also be within my power to take a life; this awesome responsibility must be faced with great humbleness and awareness of my own frailty. Above all, I must not play at God.
- I will remember that I do not treat a fever chart, a cancerous growth, but a sick human being, whose illness may affect the person's family and economic stability. My responsibility includes these related problems, if I am to care adequately for the sick.
- I will prevent disease whenever I can, for prevention is preferable to cure.
- I will remember that I remain a member of society, with special obligations to all my fellow human beings, those sound of mind and body as well as the infirm.
- If I do not violate this oath, may I enjoy life and art, respected while I live and remembered with affection thereafter.

May I always act so as to preserve the finest traditions of my calling and may I long experience the joy of healing those who seek my help.

Principlism – principles of medical ethics

In 1979, two philosophers, Beauchamp and Childress, proposed in their book *Principles of biomedical ethics*[7] an ethical approach called *principlism,* based on core ethical principles rather than ideologies of tradition, culture or religion. Many consider this work to be the standard theoretical guidelines for practising doctors to focus on moral reasoning and analyse ethical situations.

Principlism is based on four *core principles* accepted by most intellectual, cultural and religious traditions:

1. *autonomy*, the patient's right to self-determination
2. *beneficence*, the duty to do good to patients, in taking actions that serve their best interests
3. *non-maleficence*, the obligation to avoid doing harm to patients, as stated in the Hippocratic Oath, and
4. *justice*, or *distributive justice*, the fair allocation of medical resources to treat similar patients in similar ways.

These four core principles include four *core behavioural norms* to guide ethical decision making when working with patients and professional colleagues:

- *fidelity,* the duty to commit to patients, such as with advocacy, dedication, fairness and loyalty
- *confidentiality,* the duty to prevent the disclosure of private information of patients without their authorisation – as confidentiality is the glue that bonds the trust of the patient in the patient–doctor relationship
- *veracity*, the duty to provide truthful, objective and comprehensive information to patients, and
- *privacy*, the duty to respect patients' and families' rights to keep personal information and activities under their own control.

Codes of conduct for doctors

Ethics are central to every branch of medicine. *Codes of conduct* are professional policies of medical bodies such as the Australian Medical Association. These codes incorporate principles of medical ethics in caring for patients and their families, as well as principles of behavioural conduct in professional practice. As a corollary, medical professional misconduct includes undertaking any illegal activity (such as illegal abortions), negligent care, relationships – especially sexual – with patients, fake research, fraudulent records, conflicts of interest and bad-mouthing colleagues behind their backs. The case of Dr Andrew Wakefield, the most cited author in the medical literature for fraud, is an example. Dr Wakefield, a British gastroenterologist, published a research paper in the prestigious journal *The Lancet* in 1998[8] that reported a link between the administration of the measles, mumps and rubella (MMR) vaccine and the appearance of autism and inflammatory bowel disease in 12 children. Other researchers could not reproduce this result. In 2004, he was found to have undisclosed financial conflicts of interest. A General Medical Council (GMC) investigation found elements of his work to be falsified and that he had acted without prior ethical approval. *The Lancet* retracted his paper noting that it was 'utterly false', with no causal link between MMR and autism. Investigation of his raw data showed that the children had no bowel disease. The GMC struck him off the UK medical register. Despite this, fear of this link to autism and bowel disease led to a decline in MMR vaccination in UK and the US, and a corresponding rise in measles and mumps with serious illness and deaths. Dr Wakefield has continued to claim his innocence, and, unfortunately, the anti-vaccination lobby continues today to discourage parents from vaccinating their children.

*

Jason Black, the patient in question, was an obese, big, barrel-chested man sitting upright in bed, wheezing and breathing with difficulty and wearing a mask-ventilation circuit. His lips were blue and he had thick, nicotine-stained fingers that contrasted with his bluish nail beds. He could not speak and occasionally coughed up and dribbled foul-smelling sputum into a bowl, which necessitated removal of his facemask. The technique of mask-ventilation uses a tight-fitting facemask connected to a special ventilator. The ventilator assists breathing with in-breaths triggered by the patient's own spontaneous inspiration, which is far less efficient than conventional ventilation through a tracheal tube. Gas leaks around the mask and some is forced into the stomach. Patients find mask-ventilation claustrophobic and uncomfortable, but it can buy time for recovery and avoids difficult or failed weaning because the trachea is not intubated. Often it is unsuccessful in advanced COPD, as it was with Jason Black. Two days after admission, his condition deteriorated and we had to decide whether to intubate his trachea. Following discussions among us and with Dr Will Mullins, head of respiratory medicine, the decision was a resounding 'No'. I was to discuss this with his family.

Jason Black was a widower. His three sons, aged in their thirties, were standing in the interview room when I walked in. They ran the family trucking business started by their father. All three had dark curly hair and the same body shape, big and burly, like New

Zealand's All Blacks rugby forwards. They even dressed the same, in checked lumberjack shirts, jeans and steel-capped work boots. Rachel then walked in. They could not take their eyes off this young, attractive Eurasian doctor. I sensed her unease as she sidestepped to be almost behind me. They stared ominously in silence and we remained standing. No one offered to shake hands. They radiated aggression and hostility. In the front was the eldest and Jason Black's substitute decision maker, the leader I remembered from the last admission. He was the only one with a sprinkling of grey hair. *How do I start this?* I wondered, but number one son could not contain himself any longer. 'When you gonna fix him then?', he said in a gruff voice.

'I'm afraid I've got bad news', I said. 'Your father is dying. He's not responding to treatment.'

'What do you mean? You can put him on the machine, the respirator, like last time, you know.'

'No. He's reached the end stage of his lung disease. The ventilator will not save him this time.'

'How would you know? You're not putting him on the respirator?', he hissed. His eyes widened. 'You're still blaming his smoking again?'

'His lungs are now far too damaged. We're trying our best but ... I'm sorry; the sad news is that he is slipping away, regardless of what we do. Ventilation will only delay his passing for a few days. It's futile and risky and would cause him too much suffering ... not in his best interests.' I tried to calm his gathering wrath.

'Risky? He did OK last time. He can't die. Suffering? He's a real fighter. I'm telling you, we want him on the respirator. *He needs full treatment!*' His lips curled in determination and anger. He turned round to his brothers as the lead wolf of the pack. 'He's got a right to smoke too, you know. It's his body.'

I did not comment on his last point, one that all smokers make. That arose because we had previously strongly advised his father to stop smoking. Of course, every person has the right to smoke but when – not if – they succumb to serious diseases that smoking inflicts, they expect the state, the taxpayer, to fund their healthcare that is needed from exercising that right to smoke.

They moved menacingly closer. Number one son's face blackened. 'We'll report you, you know, if you don't use the machine. Are you docs doing euthanasia? Bad for you, you know.' *Is that a threat?* I thought. After that outburst, I could see no benefit in prolonging our meeting, and I shepherded Rachel out. It was one of the worst family discussions I have had. Perhaps I could have handled it better, but they were projecting their concerns for their father as blame on the carers. They were angrily demanding futile treatment. And they were physically intimidating.

Jason Black died the next day, with his sons at his bedside. Initially belligerent, they settled down and were, in the end, decent to the nurses. Nonetheless, they lodged formal complaints to the hospital and their local politician about our professional lack of care. Their claims were rejected after official reviews. We had decided not to institute futile mechanical ventilation in Jason Black's best interests, as that would not have saved his life but would have inappropriately prolonged his suffering. We chose *beneficence* and *distributive justice* over *autonomy*, the demands made by his family. Jason Black chose not to stop smoking. In a way, this was how he chose how to die.

*

Hierarchy of ethical principles in clinical decision making

In the Hippocratic Oath the primary principle is *primum non nocere* – 'first, do no harm' – the principle of *non-maleficence*, an axiom taught to medical students. Some bioethicists have challenged this, arguing instead for the primary principle to be *autonomy*. Different people also argue for different ethical hierarchies. Others argue for the application of all the relevant principles to each case, with the clinical scenario determining the hierarchy of importance. There have been studies of philosophical questions on the nature, validity and usefulness of the four core principles (and others as well), often using medical students as subjects. In general, participants were able to identify ethical issues consistent with the principles in the theoretical clinical cases they were presented with.[9] However, different stakeholders identified the nature of the principles differently, and there were difficulties with applying them to hypothetical cases. Females valued autonomy more than males, and medical students were in general more beneficent than lawyers.[10] One study showed a significant preference for *non-maleficence* over the other three.[11]

However, although some participants recognised the value of ethical principles, they did not use them directly in decision making in hypothetical clinical cases. This suggested that, in the real world, doctors may not base decisions on abstract ethical principles but rather respond cognitively only to the unique clinical scenario. Hence, how healthcare professionals apply ethical principles in decision making cannot be deduced from research literature. Nonetheless, all principles are important and must be respected, and clinicians must always consider their patient's best interests.

Ethics in end-of-life care

Ethics guide doctors in making decisions related to death and dying. However, medical ethics and codes of conduct will not always provide simple straightforward answers. Some doctors may feel unfocused by the complexities of moral arguments, and hence be unsure how to address the presenting complicated, urgent ethical issue. Nonetheless, healthcare professionals must be cognisant of the principles to address issues that confront them, their patients and their families at the end of life.

With *patient autonomy,* communication about end-of-life care and use of advance care directives with the patient and family is important. Awareness of the principle can be preserved even if the patient loses the capacity to make decisions.

With *beneficence*, doctors must do what they believe is in the patient's best interests, but while respecting the patient's right to self-determination. However, in some clinical situations, the judged best interests of the patient can conflict with the patient's preferences (see later in this chapter).

With *non-maleficence*, decisions must not knowingly inflict harm to the patient. This principle can be breached by the *doctrine of double effect* – that is, if a therapeutic treatment has a bad side effect, giving that treatment is justified as the bad effect was not intended. However, helping the patient to self-harm violates this principle. Many view doctor-assisted suicide or euthanasia as such a breach of ethics.

With *justice*, doctors should advocate for just and equitable treatment of their dying patients without discrimination.

With *veracity* and *fidelity*, doctors should be truthful to their dying patients regarding the diagnosis, prognosis and treatment plans. This full disclosure may not be the preference in some cultures and with some families.

Some of the most difficult issues in medical ethics today arise from conflicts with *autonomy*. The costs of healthcare, particularly expensive technology that sustain life, are high. Dilemmas arise when *autonomy* conflicts with *distributive justice*. Use of valuable, expensive resources in futile, full-blown treatment in cases similar to Jason Black's contravenes this principle. On a personal level, in acting for the patient's best interests, *beneficence* may conflict with *autonomy*. Patients and families may disagree with the treatments that healthcare professionals recommend in their best interests. Western medicine, in general, supports the wishes of a mentally competent person, but other cultures and societies may prioritise *beneficence* over *autonomy* ('doctor knows best'). In some circumstances, the state's interest in the preservation of life may override *autonomy* to enforce a course of treatment. Hence, issues in advance care directives (Chapter 3), distributive justice (Chapter 16), confidentiality, futile medical care including withdrawing or withholding life-sustaining treatment (Chapter 6) and 'do not resuscitate' (DNR) orders (Chapter 4), arise in end-of-life care. These issues are discussed in their specific chapters. The ethical and legal principle of informed consent (Chapter 8), however, can never be bypassed.

Reflections

- There are potential ethical dilemmas in end-of-life care.
- Doctors should be cognisant of these dilemmas and communicate accordingly with the patient and family.
- Decisions regarding treatment are guided by ethical principles, but with the patient's best interests foremost in mind. Beneficence and distributive justice then take precedence over autonomy.
- Effective communication is vital.

References

1. The Ad Hoc Committee of the Harvard Medical School to Examine the Definition of Death. A definition of irreversible coma. *JAMA* 1968;205:337.
2. Kübler-Ross E. *On death and dying.* New York: Macmillan; 1969.

3. Australian Institute of Health and Welfare. *Australian Burden of Disease Study 2015: Interactive data on disease burden.* Australian Burden of Disease Cat. no. BOD 24. Canberra, ACT: AIHW; 2019.

4. Australian Institute of Health and Welfare. *Disease expenditure in Australia.* HWE no. 76. Canberra, ACT: AIHW; 2019. https://aihw.gov.au.

5. Shavelle RM, Paculdo DR, Kush SJ, Mannino DM, Strauss DJ. Life expectancy and years of life lost in chronic obstructive pulmonary disease: findings from the NHANES III follow-up study. *Int J Chronic Obstr Pulm Dis* 2009;4:137–48.

6. Lasagna L. The revised Hippocratic Oath. www.doctors.practo.com.

7. Beauchamp TL, Childress JF. *Principles of biomedical ethics.* New York: Oxford University Press; 1979; 8th ed. 2019.

8. Wakefield AJ, Murch SH, Anthony A, Linnell J, Casson DM, Malik M, et al. Ileal lymphoid nodular hyperplasia, non-specific colitis, and pervasive developmental disorder in children [retracted]. *Lancet* 1998;351:637–41.

9. Herbert PC, Meslin EM, Dunn EV. Measuring the ethical sensitivity of medical students: a study at the University of Toronto. *J Med Ethics* 1992;18(3):142–7.

10. Schwartz R, Rezler AG, Lambert P, Obenshein SS, Gibson JM, Bennahum DA. Professional decisions and ethical values in medical and law students. *Acad Med* 1990;65:31–2.

11. Page K. The four principles: can they be measured and do they predict ethical decision-making? *BMC Med Ethics* 2012;13:10.

3

Advance care directives

Telling how you choose to die

This I choose to do. If there is a price, this I choose to pay. If it is my death, then I choose to die. Where this takes me, there I choose to go. I choose. This I choose to do.

Terry Pratchet (1948–2015), English author, in *Wintersmith* (2006)[1]

*

An *advance care directive* (ACD) is also known as an *advance health directive* or colloquially as a 'living will'. It is a legal document or statement completed by a competent adult that prescribes his or her preferences for future medical treatment if he or she loses capacity to make such decisions. Preferences recorded in an ACD are significant considerations in end-of-life care.

*

'The ICU doctors asked us if Nana had a *living will*. A living will, Tom! I thought it existed only in America, on TV … like *House MD* shows!' My neighbour Mike was telling me about his grandmother's admission to hospital with a massive stroke. The doctors had enquired about his grandmother's ACD.

'I suppose you doctors must hate living wills. They tie your hands in treating patients, don't they? Having to legally comply with wishes pre-death? What if they are unreasonable, impractical, even illegal?'

*

Scope of advance care directives

An ACD may cover only refusals of treatment, or it may encompass options for care, with or without nominating a person to make decisions on the patient's behalf. This surrogate is known as a *healthcare proxy* or *substitute decision maker*. An ACD is based on the patient's autonomy to receive care and to die in accordance with their values, and need not be limited to end-of-life decisions. It is a component of an *advance care plan* (Chapter 4 Do not resuscitate) and should not be confused with a resuscitation plan or a clinical treatment plan. It covers only healthcare and no handling of assets. ACDs in Australia have a high level of variability though a standard national format has been proposed.[2] In the ICU, ACDs have more acute emphases than those in nursing homes or hospital wards as death is quick if life-sustaining treatment is stopped.

Laws on ACD identify a substitute decision maker to make decisions for the incapacitated patient. If no ACD is in place, the substitute decision maker is recognised to be a family member, according to an established hierarchy[a] or, where applicable, a state-appointed adult guardian. A substitute decision maker is expected to make substituted decisions that the patient would have made. If there is no applicable preference in the ACD, the substitute decision maker decides in the person's best interests according to the patient's values, goals and beliefs. The substitute decision maker can consent to or refuse treatment offered, but cannot demand treatment.

An ACD can also be an oral statement made by the patient to the healthcare team, and it should be recorded in the patient's notes. The legal validity of a 'conversational' oral statement made

---

[a] In most jurisdictions, the order is spouse or *de facto*, adult children, adult siblings.

by the patient to family or friends that was unwritten but later recalled from memory has not been tested in an Australian court. Its relevance could be decided in the hospital without necessarily raising problems as, arguably, oral statements have always been an integral part of medical practice.

Origins of advance care directives

ACDs can claim roots from the 1960s, when life-prolonging treatments were improved (e.g. cardiopulmonary resuscitation, CPR) or pioneered (e.g. care in ICUs). Increasing community concerns regarding patient advocacy drove new laws such as legislation on 'living wills'. In the US in the late 1970s, the case of Karen Quinlan – a young woman with irrecoverable, severe brain damage (Chapter 6 Withdrawing treatment) – drew attention to the ethical and legal dilemmas raised by incompetent patients receiving life support. Her parents went to court wanting to disconnect the ventilator from their daughter, but her doctors vigorously opposed their application. A decade later, the Nancy Cruzan case (Chapter 6 Withdrawing treatment) repeated the legal battle between the state's interest to preserve life and what an incompetent patient would want, as expressed by their family. This case resulted in the US Congress passing the *Patient Self-Determination Act* to promote ACDs on a national level. In the 1980s and 1990s, Australia established recognition of ACDs and substitute decision makers in common law and statutory law in some states, and in 2011 introduced a National Framework to standardise common goals.[2] Similarly, the UK's *Mental Capacity Act 2005* and New Zealand's *Bill of Rights Act 1990* respect the stated rights of incompetent adult individuals to refuse medical treatment.

*

'Dr Benson's seen him. He had nothing to add', Josh Shaw said. I stood beside bed 11 with Josh, Paul Constable and Rachel Lim. Dr Benson was a general surgeon who had performed bariatric gastric sleeve surgery on the patient in bed 11. The procedure, by 'keyhole' laparoscopic surgery, was to enable a morbidly obese, 45-year-old John Coolup to lose weight. This removes 80% of the stomach, leaving a banana-shaped 'sleeve' joining the oesophagus to the small intestines. The much smaller stomach results in feelings of fullness sooner, and ultimately in long-term weight loss. Sleeve gastrectomies are generally safe and effective, but staple line leaks are serious postoperative complications and the incidence can exceed 2%; mortality is rare at less than 0.2%.[2]

John Coolup was unfortunately one of the rare complications. His staple line leak had resulted in peritonitis and septicaemia unresponsive to antibiotics. He consequently developed the condition called adult respiratory distress syndrome (ARDS). The major characteristic of ARDS is diffuse damage of the lungs with the release of inflammatory chemicals that cause shock and impair functioning of organs. Multiorgan failure heralded his downward, irreversible spiral into the 'twilight zone'.

John Coolup lay in bed, with his back raised, heavily sedated, intubated and ventilated, and decked with the usual ICU monitoring and IV lines. Two large tubes into his abdomen drained a dark greenish-yellow fluid, flecked with spots of black. His urine catheter showed concentrated, dark urine. The ventilator delivered a high oxygen concentration, but his oxygenation indices were poor.

Paul shook his head. 'Not good news', he said in an understatement. He bent down to examine the urine collection bag. 'Urine volume's falling.' He straightened up to look at the blood chemistry results on the charts. 'I see that his coags are heading downhill as well.' Paul referred to Mr Coolup's coagulation or blood-clotting results. Clotting disorders (coagulopathy) are part of the manifestations of multiorgan failure. Mr Coolup had been in the ICU for three weeks now. We had given him optimal treatment for his ARDS, but his lungs and kidneys had deteriorated and now, with his coagulopathy, multiorgan failure had become a reality.

'Question is – do we start dialysis?', I said. The two registrars shook their heads. The mortality rate for ARDS is 40%–60%, and much higher with sepsis, morbid obesity and the severity of signs displayed by Mr Coolup.

'Let's see what develops over the next couple of days. We should consult the renal people', Paul said.

'Agreed. And I'll talk with Mrs Coolup', I said.

The renal physicians saw Mr Coolup and, as we suspected, agreed with our bleak prognosis and declined to institute dialysis. Over the next two days, his condition worsened further.

I saw Mrs Coolup in the interview room. She came alone without their two teenage daughters. Jane Coolup was as petite as her husband was big, and poised and well dressed in a black business suit. She was also a lawyer, a partner in a different firm to her husband's. I had previously discussed ARDS with her and I updated her with his condition, ending up with the findings of the renal physicians. With this intelligent lady, I didn't couch my words in reassuring or imprecise terms.

'Jane, as you know the mortality of ARDS is high. With a smoking history, high blood pressure and morbid obesity, mortality from ARDS secondary to sepsis from a bowel leak is much higher. And John has these extra factors', I said.

'How high?' she asked.

'Mortality? We think at this stage, over 90%. He now has four organ systems in failure – lungs, bowels, blood clotting and kidneys. His heart is failing too, struggling to maintain his blood pressure. At this stage, he needs kidney dialysis. The renal physicians will not proceed unless we push them.'

'Do you think he has a chance? No matter how small?', she asked, with no hint of anxiety in her voice.

'In my view and those of my colleagues, no.' I gave her a brief account of prognostications in critical illness with examples of similar multiorgan failure cases we have had.

'He has an advance care directive, you know', she said matter-of-factly, which raised my eyebrows. Neither she nor Dr Benson had mentioned it before. 'He made it before his surgery. He consented to, and wanted, intensive care, ventilation, CPR *and dialysis.*' She spoke clearly as I imagined she would in court, but her trembling left hand (which she steadied by gripping her knee), betrayed her calm demeanour.

'He might not have anticipated a situation as grave as this', I said. 'If he did, what would he have wanted? *In his best interests …?* What would you want for him?'

Her self-control cracked briefly. I saw tears glistening before she quickly looked down. She took a deep breath, blinked and regained her composure. 'I think I … John … would not want dialysis', she said softly. I nodded. I had the feeling that she had been thinking about this the past few days. No doubt she would have researched ARDS, multiorgan failure, futile treatment and withdrawal of treatment, with the Australian and US cases tested in court. She then stood up, thanked me with a sad smile, shook my hand and, with grace and dignity, departed. I learnt later that her specialty was litigation law. I hoped Dr Benson's medical indemnity insurance was up to date.

We did not proceed to dialysis, but we did not withdraw treatment. John Coolup died two days later, a week from his 46th birthday, with Jane and their daughters at his bedside. He had an ACD to proceed to dialysis that we did not follow because that was futile care and not in his best interests.

*

Advance care directives and the law

Many countries now require healthcare institutions to provide information to patients on how to complete ACDs to record their preferences for appropriate care, including end-of-life care. ACDs are based on the principle of patient autonomy – your right to direct the care of your future incapacitated self. True, there are advantages. An ACD can help clarify your values, beliefs and wishes for end-of-life care. Conflict between and within all parties – your family and your doctors – can often be avoided during the dying process, when strong emotions can hamper decision making. Better end-of-life care and family satisfaction have been reported, with less anxiety, stress and depression experienced by family members. However, there are disadvantages too as we shall see. About 10% of ACDs are completed near death, 30% when chronically ill and 60% when well.[3] In the US less than 10% of the population have ACDs, and the percentage in Australia is 14%.

The legal status of ACDs varies between countries, but if legislated they are binding on doctors. Common to all ACDs are these basic principles: the patient was competent when they made an ACD, the directive was intended for the current situation, and the patient was not pressured into making it. In Australia, ACD is a collective term to describe legislated and common law instruments to respect self-determined preferences for healthcare, but not for legal or financial matters. The right to autonomy requires that the wishes of a competent adult be respected, and treatment not be given contrary to that directive. However, the law recognises that there are appropriate circumstances in which a health professional should be excused from following an ACD.

These relate to preferences that are illegal, or considered futile, unwarranted or medically inappropriate. Also, directives need not be followed if based on a misunderstanding of available treatments, or where circumstances have changed significantly since the directive was made. These were considered by Jane Coolup in her decision not to insist on dialysis for her husband. He was not aware of, or had not anticipated, terminal multiorgan failure when he made his ACD. Luke Bannon, in the following case, is another example of the law's acceptance of a present-time *contemporaneous substituted judgment* to overlook a refusal of treatment in his ACD.

*

Josh, Wesley and I were resuscitating a new male patient in bed 15. Josh inserted three vascular lines, and Wesley intubated him and then connected him to the ventilator. Jacinta, the bed nurse, had secured his monitoring cables and was about to insert a urine catheter. Mr Luke Bannon was an obese 40-year-old with insulin-dependent diabetes mellitus, brought to the emergency department in a diabetic ketoacidosis coma. He had an angry-looking infection on his right toe.

'I put his wife in the interview room. She's waiting for you', Jacinta said.

Jody Bannon looked younger than fortyish, with short dark hair. She glanced up as I entered, her eyes misted and wide with worry. Luke was a heavy-machinery salesman, she told me, having had to travel extensively away from home in the past three weeks. It was likely that dehydration, poor eating and disordered insulin use from his travels gave rise to the diabetic coma, triggered by his toe infection. I explained his condition, how we had resuscitated him and what we were going to do.

She fidgeted in her chair and looked away. Her troubled face, with her eyebrows drawn together, suggested serious concerns for her husband. She bit her lower lip before blurting out, 'He's got a living will.'

'That's good. What does it say? Have you got it here?', I said, surprised. I strangely felt relieved although I did not know what to expect.

She dug nervously into her bag and drew out a document. It was a run-of-the-mill form titled 'living will', available from some newsagents. The handwritten entries made by Luke Bannon appeared valid, but I noted his *refusal* under *treatment decisions* for 'intensive care', 'life support' and 'mechanical ventilation'.

She saw the frown on my face and said, 'He doesn't want to depend on me. He knows he can go into diabetic coma and doesn't want to end up a ... a *vegetable* if resuscitated. He doesn't want intensive care and not on the ventilator and life support to be left a vegetable.'

Apparently his fear came from seeing his uncle who was incapacitated from a stroke. I explained to her that Luke would die if his diabetic coma were left untreated. With treatment, he had more than a 90% chance of survival without incapacitation, but treatment must involve intensive care and ventilation. 'Jody, the law allows us to disregard Luke's living will if it is inappropriate, which it is. We will continue with our treatment, but it would be good if you do not disagree.'

She twisted the handkerchief in her hands, with a pinched-looking face, torn between being loyal to his wishes and being disloyal to save him. I thought she was about to burst into tears when she said, 'Save him please.'

We continued with Luke Bannon's treatment. He recovered, left the ICU five days later, and was discharged home after another week. A month later, he and Jody came to see us, bearing gifts. He had lost weight and looked to be in good health. 'Thank God you didn't follow my living will', he said. 'I'm a machinery salesman. I'd be pushing up daisies and John Deere tractors by now.'

*

In Luke's case, the state's interest in the preservation of life reasonably requires a directive to be disregarded if there is a valid contemporaneous substituted judgment. Luke made a choice to refuse life support because he had misconceptions about intensive care treatment. He did not die because we did not follow his choice. If we had, we would have paradoxically failed to respect his autonomy to put his best interests first. A healthy person and a future same, but sick and incompetent, person are two different persons. We make choices when we are well, but when we become sick our values and priorities may change in the course of the illness. The present person tends to *underestimate* their will to live, and *overestimate* their emotional burden, should they become incapacitated in the future. People with physical or chronic disability often show a zest for living, reporting happiness and a good quality of life despite all odds – a concept called '*disability paradox*' or '*hedonic adaptation*'. The onset of their illness or disability causes them distress which becomes long term if the condition continually worsens or is associated with pain and severe discomfort. If the illness or disability does not get worse, they adjust to their new condition and consider themselves to be reasonably happy. I have seen patients in hospital who recovered with such inspiring qualities despite some residual disabilities. As a corollary, I have never encountered a patient harbouring any regrets that his or her life was saved. Also, from my experience, not every patient prizes autonomy. Some prefer their doctors or family members to decide for them, and others have cultural reservations about discussing their end-of-life care (Chapter 13 Cultures and ethnicities).

What happens should a family and the doctors strongly disagree on the preferences in an ACD? Hospitals have, or should have, policies and guidelines to resolve this. The process involves discussions among the two parties, independent specialists and hospital ethicists. Determining what is in the patient's best interests must be the primary objective. Going to court should be the last resort.

Problems with advance care directives

ACDs may pose potential problems. A major one is epistemic – a limited capacity for any individual to imagine future scenarios and use words to predict *every* potential condition or circumstance which *may or may not occur*. To exclude or reject treatments termed 'life support' or 'life sustaining' in an ACD can be counterproductive. Almost every intervention in the ICU, from complex invasive procedures like ventilation and kidney dialysis to routine practices like infusing fluids, can be considered measures to support or sustain life. I can't know which intervention I should not use in an ACD that refuses treatment described in those general terms. On the other hand, too-detailed instructions can 'railroad' interpretations of wishes. Either way, misconceptions can inadvertently cause conflict with good clinical care. ACDs also need to clarify subtleties in scenarios – such as cognitive versus physical 'impairment', degrees of pain suffering and probable versus negligible chance of survival – as preferences will vary accordingly.

Outcome-based ACDs that express a person's values, goals, preferred quality of life and medical outcomes sought should provide more clarity than simply listing medical interventions. People also may change their medical treatment preferences owing to new experiences or priorities over time, but fail to update their ACDs.

Doctors' attitudes towards end-of-life care may be influenced by their culture, ethnicity and gender, which may impact on their *interpretation* of preferences in ACDs. It is not surprising that doctors' treatments are sometimes viewed by families as anything from overzealous to neglectful. Similarly, decisions of a substitute decision maker may not be accurate appraisals of the patient's wishes. The substitute decision maker may be confused by legalities and principles of the ACD. They may project their own values, and even dismiss preferences to favour treatment, perceiving it to be in the patient's best interest.

A large US study[4] showed that ACDs had no significant effect on limiting resuscitation efforts at time of death. Many ACDs do not explicitly state preferences for resuscitation such as a wish for a 'do not resuscitate' order. They are sometimes too vague to be relevant or to give useful information about the patient's wishes. Also, many people do not want their future treatment to be determined by previously written documents. Living wills cannot and do not resolve many dilemmas about how 'aggressive' treatment should be at the end of life.

*

Reflections

- Everyone should make an ACD that should be clear about preferences.
- Illegal, inappropriate, vague or all-encompassing requests are unhelpful.
- An ACD should nominate a substitute decision maker and be reviewed periodically.
- Medical decisions place prime significance on the patient's best interests. When in acute end-of-life situations, patient *autonomy* in an ACD may conflict with *beneficence* and *distributive justice* principles.
- Doctors need not follow an ACD that is illegal or considered futile, unwarranted, medically inappropriate or not contemporary.

References

1. Pratchett T. *Wintersmith*. New York: Harper Teen; 2006.
2. Lim R, Beekley A, Johnson DC, Davis KA. Early and late complications of bariatric operation. *Trauma Surg Acute Care Open* 2018;3(1):e000219.
3. Australian Health Ministers Advisory Council. *National framework for advance care directives*. Canberra, ACT: AHMAC; 2011.
4. The SUPPORT Principal Investigators. A controlled trial to improve care for seriously ill hospitalized patients. The study to understand prognoses and preferences for outcomes and risks of treatments (SUPPORT). *JAMA* 1995;274:1591.

Futility

4

Do not resuscitate

End of the line

Judge Winter: 'The DNR order was witnessed by Doctor House's own staff ... a Doctor Foreman.'
Dr Gregory House: 'My staff are idiots.'

House MD, TV series, in 'DNR', a 2005 episode

*

A DNR means a 'do not resuscitate' order. It means the same as 'DNAR' (do not attempt resuscitation) or 'NFR' (not for resuscitation). DNR orders instruct staff not to undertake cardiopulmonary resuscitation (CPR) if the patient's breathing stops or if the heart stops beating. Such orders are common and significant in end-of-life care.

*

Josh Shaw walked into the ICU, slightly breathless and red faced. Sweat stained his shirt and coated his forehead; he was literally hot under the collar.

'What's wrong?', I asked.

'Bloody shambles', he said. He shook his head, jaws clenched, and recounted his experience. 'I rushed to ward 6 to answer a code blue. Started CPR on Mrs Snooks, an oldie in a single room.

I intubated her while the RMO, Dr Mary Jenkins, did cardiac massage. We managed to get her ticker going, and she started to breathe. She was 73 years old, Mary told me, with colon Ca stage 2,[a] under Dr Benson, and they were prepping her for surgery next week. Mary had no idea why she arrested: history of angina, nothing serious. While I was listening to her chest, the charge nurse, Sue – who had been in a meeting – rushed in and stopped everyone, saying "DNR, Dr Patel's orders". There was no such notice in the room. Mary rifled through the medical notes; nothing there either and Patel hadn't told her. Sue said that it was mentioned in the nursing handover – tried to blame the poor bed nurse, who looked like shit. She had just started her shift and in the heat of the moment, I guess, forgot what she was told at handover. No one knew where that idiot Patel was. Mary threw up her hands in disgust, really pissed off. I extubated the patient, who was still unconscious. Told Sue to inform Benson and the Snooks family and left.'

*

DNR – do not resuscitate order

A DNR order applies to identified patients for whom cardio-pulmonary arrest would be an expected terminal event, and in whom CPR would be inappropriate. A DNR order applies only to CPR. It does not mean 'no further treatment'. All other treatment and care, especially palliative and end-of-life care, will continue for the patient. DNR decisions should be incorporated into a patient's *advance care plan* (ACP, see later in this chapter), and also a *resuscitation plan* that some hospitals use.

In common law, the patient has to give consent for the medical treatment to proceed, except in cases of emergency. The common law of necessity allows treatment in emergencies in the best interests of the patient – in this case CPR – if there is no DNR or advance care directive (ACD) that refuses resuscitation. In doctor shows on TV, miraculous survivals following CPR are almost universal. In reality, from various studies, 16%–44% survive the initial in-hospital resuscitation, and only 3%–16% survive to

---

[a]   Large bowel cancer (colon) that has not spread outside the bowel wall.

hospital discharge. Less than 4% of those with chronic, debilitating illness survive. Figures for out-of-hospital cardiac arrests are far worse. Furthermore, consequences from CPR include rib fractures, prolonged ICU stay and brain damage in survivors. There are thus compelling reasons not to conduct CPR in the event of a cardiac arrest when deemed futile or unwanted, especially on those at the end of life.

Legality of DNR orders

There is no single national law on DNR orders in Australia, and laws regarding it are obscure with respect to names and variations. Common law covers DNR preferences stated in ACDs, as mentioned in Chapter 3. A competent patient has a right to refuse resuscitation, regardless whether they have made an ACD. Where the patient is incompetent, varying legislations in the states and territories allow for a substitute decision maker to choose.

Various Australian and other health bodies have encouraged implementation of hospital advance care plans that include DNR policies. However, large variations exist in these policies, regarding definitions of DNR, who makes them, involvement of competent patients, and documentation.[1] Many Australian hospitals do not have such policies or guidelines, a situation also reported in many countries. This is a concern as doctors and nurses differ in their perception of DNR orders. Also, many policies do not address disagreements within the medical team or between the doctor and the patient or family. A good policy should address these issues, be clear and concise, and apply to the hospital setting and local cultural norms. There should be a system for review, as the patient may improve to negate the DNR order, resuscitation being no longer considered futile. The presence of a policy does not circumvent legal and ethical difficulties, or guarantee it will be followed, if the staff members are unaware of its contents. Respecting the wishes of the patient is then at risk.

*

Josh Shaw wiped his forehead as he continued to tell me his story of the code blue cardiopulmonary arrest in ward 6. He took a breath and said, 'Next thing I knew, when I had walked to the lifts, the bloody pager went off again. Same ward 6. I ran there and Sue told me that Benson had revoked Patel's DNR over the phone, and the lady had arrested again. This time we couldn't get the old biddy going', he finished, shaking his head with a sigh.

Dr Ryan Patel, the protagonist in Josh's saga, was a young British Indian surgeon who had moved from London to Australia with his wife at the start of the year. He was London born and enjoyed the trappings of a wealthy family – private school, university and a beautiful Australian wife. A man not given to humility, he had always viewed his station in life generally, and as a surgeon particularly, as being celestial. Professionally, he was monumentally obnoxious, attracting complaints from sundry patients and staff. The Royal Australasian College of Surgeons had deemed his British training and qualification as 'not comparable' to their Fellowship, requiring him to complete another year's training in Australia. To him, it was a racist cross to bear. Without discussing with anyone, not even his boss, Dr Benson, he gave a verbal DNR order on Mrs Snooks to the bed nurse. He did not fill in the standard hospital DNR form, and he did not record the instruction in the medical notes as required. When the charge nurse rang Dr Benson after the first CPR episode, he blew his top and revoked the DNR order.

*

DNR order – responsibility and consent

The responsibility to initiate a DNR order rests with the most senior doctor in charge of the patient's care, who should be cognisant of the patient's wishes and the view of other staff members and the patient's family. In Mrs Snooks's case, that was her consultant, Dr Benson.

The legal requirement to obtain informed consent to issue a DNR order is unclear. A DNR order will respect the wish in an ACD *not* to receive CPR. However, a directive to *demand* CPR does not mandate resuscitation, if considered futile for that patient. The argument that a DNR order requires consent champions the principle of autonomy, a right to decide one's own resuscitation. However, if a patient then refuses to consent to a DNR order, his doctors may feel compelled to perform CPR when his condition deteriorates – a 'legally safer' position – despite believing treatment to be futile and not in his best interests. Most patients and families lack the medical knowledge to understand what CPR is. Patients' families commonly misconstrue CPR as a choice between life and death. They may then expect CPR, if performed, to resurrect the patient from dying albeit with his serious illness uncured. In that frame of mind, they see choosing DNR as letting the patient die, with implications of moral guilt. Many doctors still argue that unilateral DNR orders are justifiable, as their professional, unbiased perceptions are the more applicable, based on their experience, knowledge and the opinion of their peers. Some avoid DNR conversations, owing partly to their own discomfort with end-of-life discussions. Few patients proactively make unapproached DNR decisions.

Most guidelines on DNR recommend that an order should not be issued without the involvement of the patient (or the substitute decision maker if applicable) plus senior medical and nursing staff. The Australian and New Zealand Committee on Resuscitation does not support autonomous decision making.[2] 'Involvement' may be interpreted to mean discussion or implied consent and not signed informed consent, which is a different matter. Once again, good communication is key to all discussions of this nature. Discussions should provide comprehensive and clear information that may dispel inappropriate assumptions on both sides. Patients and families should be made aware of the benefits and burdens of CPR. A DNR order does not mean stopping treatment, and does not preclude other supportive measures. At the bedside, doctors and nurses have an important role in assessing the validity of a DNR order: who made the order, for what reasons, what discussion has taken place with the patient or substitute decision maker, where is it documented and if it is signed by the doctor in charge. Interestingly, if an unconscious patient presents with a skin 'do not resuscitate' tattoo, doctors can choose to ignore it as it is not a legal document. DNR decisions should be incorporated in advance care plans.

Advance care plans

An advance care plan (ACP) is the end product of *advance care planning*, an ongoing process with the patient, family and health professionals which formulates the progressing healthcare of the patient.[3] The ACP records the patient's preferences about health and personal care and treatment goals. However, unlike an ACD, an ACP is more holistic and may be made by, with or for the individual. Advance care planning may take place at any time, and usually when the patient has a serious illness. An ACP often includes a *resuscitation plan* or a preference for a DNR order.

*

In the medical audit meeting of Mrs Snooks, Dr Patel coolly maintained his right to make a DNR order. She had cancer and, at her age, resuscitation would be inappropriate. He considered himself as an experienced surgeon, able to make decisions like this one, which was ethical in his view. He acknowledged that his consultant should have been the person to make the order, but Dr Benson was operating at a private hospital and was therefore unavailable. No one had drawn his attention to the hospital's DNR polices, all of which he was unaware of. The medical clinical director resolved to follow-up educational measures for Dr Patel. Dr Benson drew criticism for not keeping a tighter rein on his unpredictable junior. As for Mrs Snooks, she might not have chosen how to die this way.

Reflections

- The medical team's leader makes a DNR order, with the information recorded and shared with the patient's family and staff members.
- Patients and families in end-of-life care should formalise an ACP that includes an ACD, resuscitation plan, preference for CPR and organ donation wishes with their doctor.

References

1. Sidhu NS, Dunkley ME, Egan MJ. "Not-for-resuscitation" orders in Australian public hospitals: policies, standardised order forms and patient information leaflets. *Med J Aust* 2007;186(2):72–5.
2. Australian and New Zealand Committee on Resuscitation. *Legal and ethical issues related to resuscitation*. Guideline 10.5. Melbourne, VIC: ANZCOR; 2015. resus.org.au.
3. NSW Health. *Advance planning for quality care at end of life*. Action plan 2013–2018. Sydney, NSW: NSW Health; 2013.

5

Prognostications
Predicting whether you die

'What could be a more negative word than "futility"?'
he said.
    'Ignorance', I said.

Kurt Vonnegut (1922–2007), American writer
in *Hocus Pocus* (1990)[1]

Tomorrow at sunrise I shall no longer be here.

Nostradamus (1503–66), French physician and oracle; said a
day before his death.

*

Prognostications in medical care mean predictions of patient outcomes – death or survival, and the scope of the survivor's physical and cognitive abilities on discharge from hospital. Predicting outcome is a potentially useful tool in treating the seriously ill: end-of-life care plans can be made if mortality is on the cards. Considerations of futility in a patient's end-of-life care require clinical assessments. Models that score severity of illness to predict outcome in individuals have a level of precision that is, well, unpredictable.

*

'Obviously the ICU doctors had decided that treatment for Nana was futile. They're not Gods, although it seems to me that some bask under that self-delusional aura. How could they be so sure?', Mike my neighbour asked, regarding his grandmother's admission to hospital with a massive stroke. The doctors had advised his family that her prognosis was dire.

*

Prognostications and futility

Every day in the hospital, doctors consider decisions to start or continue specific treatments in patients. Decision making judges the effectiveness of the treatment to achieve desired outcomes. Treatment is withheld or withdrawn if considered futile (Chapter 6 Withdrawing treatment). 'Futile treatment' or 'futility' in relation to medical care spans medicine, law and ethics, but there is no consensus in defining the term. The basic concept proposes the improbability or unlikelihood of attaining a treatment goal, such as preservation of life, a physiological state or an ascribed quality of life. A common definition is *'Treatment that no longer provides a benefit to a patient, or treatment where the burdens of treatment outweigh the benefits'.*[2] Futility is a combination of the concepts of causation, failure and repetition. Futile treatment, then, is the treatment for an effect that does not achieve that intended effect, no matter how often repeated.

*

Rachel Lim was back from the emergency department, looking upset. She was called to see an 83-year-old woman with a ruptured abdominal aortic aneurysm ('triple-A')[a] in a poor condition. This is a 'ballooning' bulge of the body's main blood vessel, due to weakness in its wall. Dr Ryan Patel, now on rotation to vascular surgery, was set on immediate surgery and he wanted to book a post-surgery ICU bed. Rachel declined, knowing that emergency surgery to repair a ruptured triple-A has a high mortality rate. In view of the patient's age, shock from severe blood loss and

---

[a]An abnormal swelling or bulge in the wall of the main artery, the aorta.

known heart disease, she could with high probability die on the operating table. Surgery would be futile, she decided, and she wanted to check with me.

She frowned and tried to slow down her breathing. 'Patel became angry. Stark raving bonkers.'

'What did Liz Rogers say?', I asked.

'She declined on grounds of futility. Patel had not even consulted Hodge.'

There are two techniques to repair a triple-A. Dr Liz Rogers, a consultant radiologist, was the expert on endovascular aneurysm repair (EVAR), a highly skilled procedure: a stent graft (tubular splint) is introduced in a groin vessel, and guided to the aneurysm to seal its walls. The alternative to EVAR is conventional open surgery through a large incision in the abdomen, as would be performed by Dr Adam Hodge the consultant vascular surgeon, Patel's new boss.

Rachel uncurled her stethoscope from her neck as if to remove the yoke of her recent bad experience. 'Then he yelled at me. "Futile surgery? What are you, Nostradamus? You're so bloody negative. Take some Prozac", and he stormed off.' Her lips curled in a sardonic smile. 'Nostradamus on Prozac?! Funny if it wasn't so pathetic and unprofessional.'

*

Predicting outcome

Healthcare today is expensive, with the greatest costs expended at the end-of-life and by the sickest, such as ICU patients. Delivery of inappropriate treatments is a poor use of valuable resources. Consequently, doctors have to make clinical decisions based on evaluations of outcomes and the required resources. Inappropriate treatments may include those that have some chance of achieving survival but which will result in poor quality of life, such as surviving in a persistent vegetative state (Chapter 9 Brain death and vegetative states).

Outcome determination considers the premorbid health status, underlying disease, severity of the acute insult and unwanted effects of treatment.[3] To help determine effectiveness of treatment, models to predict the mortality of critically ill patients have been developed (*see Box*). These predict prognosis for groups of patients ranked by severity of illness rather than for an individual.

Mortality Prediction Models

These include:
- Acute Physiologic and Chronic Health Evaluation II (APACHE II)
- Mortality Probability Model (MPM)
- Simplified Acute Physiology Score (SAPS).

These models calculate scores based on multiple variables – for example, type of admission, underlying diseases, physiological values and laboratory data. APACHE II considers the worst values during the first day, and MPM and SAPS scores reflect values within one hour of admission. As the patient's condition changes, the prognostic models require revalidation.

Accuracy is tested by *discrimination* and *calibration*. Discrimination is the ability of the model to distinguish between patients who die and those who survive. Calibration is the ability to match predicted death rates with actual deaths.

Prognostications can be expressed in one or both of two standards. A *quantitative* prediction expresses treatment outcome in probability terms (e.g. less than 10% chance of survival or less than six months of life). The *qualitative* standard evaluates probable residual disabilities and quality of life (e.g. persistent vegetative state). If the quantity of life is so short or improbable, or the quality of life is so reduced that the pain, suffering, distress and indignities of treatment outweigh the benefits, then the expensive treatment is inappropriate. Either way, despite reliance on objective medical evidence in its consideration, determination of futile or inappropriate treatment can be criticised as being subjective.

USEFULNESS OF PREDICTION MODELS

Outcome prediction models may be used in research to compare patient groups, assess ICU performance and guide resource allocation, but they are not sensitive or specific in predicting outcomes of individual patients. In predictions of futility, limiting 'futile' treatment may become a self-fulfilling prophecy; a high proportion of deaths that follow will artificially raise the mortality rate. Even if we exclude this factor, a high level of certainty in predicting individual poor outcome is not scientifically possible.[4]

Many studies in claims of medical futility are fettered by their empirical evidence and varying definitions of futility.[5] They also focus solely on mortality without predicting functional status after ICU intervention. The latter is a key issue with families regarding the patient's future quality of life and care needed. Doctors may raise these prediction models in discussions of treatment with families, but they should not use them as the sole, final or even primary determinant of futility.[6]

Doctors' and families' notions of futility

The failure to cause a desired effect or to realise a goal, as set by predetermined values, determines medical futility. By this notion, futile treatment is judged largely on how the doctor conceives of and defines the value-laden goal, which families may not accept. For example, families may regard the poor odds against survival, an extra short period of prolonged life or a reduced quality of life, as worth continuing treatment for, despite any attendant and consequential burdens on the patient and family. As the doctor's goal may be loftier than that accepted by the family, the doctor's standard is higher than the family's in judging whether treatment is effective; the higher the standard, the greater the likelihood that treatment will be considered futile. Hence, the doctor and the family can reach different conclusions about whether treatment is worthwhile.

Hospitals should have policies or guidelines in communicating with families regarding disagreements on care. Discussions should be clear on the patient's considered prognosis, what the patient's and doctors' goals are, what treatment is appropriate for, what treatment will or will not achieve and what burdens treatment will impose. Enlisting other health professionals such as other specialists or social workers is often helpful.

There are two principal ethical reasons why treatment may be classed as futile or inappropriate: *beneficence* – that it is contrary to the patient's best interests, and *distributive justice* (Chapter 16) – that it uses resources that may deny treatment to, and thus indirectly harm, other patients. The latter reasoning is controversial and should not be the primary or sole reason.

Whether treatment is considered futile is initially a matter for the treating doctors, but this decision can be challenged in court. Australian courts have employed the test of what is in the patient's interests, considering the *benefits* versus the *burden of treatment* on the patient such as unwarranted pain or indignity.

Doctors who often make treatment decisions on severely ill patients are aware of the limitations of outcome prediction models. They do not use the models in everyday work, but only as assessment tools in certain cases to complement factual clinical details. In general, ICU staff, especially nurses, agree with the medical decisions regarding inappropriate treatment, although nurses are more pessimistic in predicting outcomes.[7] The patients' families, however, tend to have a low level of confidence in doctors' abilities to prognosticate.[8] This again raises the importance of good communication and trust building by the doctors.

Rachel's 83-year-old lady with a ruptured triple-A had no realistic chance of survival from emergency surgical repair, based on our assessment and experience. I agreed with her decision to decline ICU admission. The patient received end-of-life care and died in a way that she did not choose, but without further futile, burdensome and expensive interventions.

*

Reflections

- Outcome prediction models are not used for making decisions on individual patients.
- For critically ill patients, families consider the treatment options with their doctors accordingly:
  o What are the treatment goals?
  o What are the probable quantitative and qualitative consequences of the proposed treatment?
  o What are the burdensome consequences of the treatment?
  o What are in the patient's best interests?
- Families should ask for a second opinion if unsatisfied with information provided.

References

1. Vonnegut K. *Hocus pocus*. New York: Rosetta Books; 1990.
2. Australian Medical Association. *End-of-life care and advance care planning*. Position statement. Barton, ACT: AMA; 2014. https://ama.com.au/position-statement/end-life-care-and-advance-care-planning-2014.

3. Dodek PM, Heyland DK, Rocker GM, Cook DJ. Translating family satisfaction data into quality improvement. *Crit Care Med* 2004;32(9):1922–7.
4. Wilkinson DJ, Savulescu J. Knowing when to stop: futility in the ICU. *Curr Opin Anaesthesiol* 2011;24(2):160–5.
5. Gabbay E, Calvo-Broce J, Meyer KB, Trikalinos TA, Cohen J, Kent DM. The empirical basis for determinations of medical futility. *J Gen Intern Med* 2010;25(10):1083–9.
6. Mendez-Tellez PA, Dorman T. Predicting patient outcomes, futility, and resource utilization in the Intensive Care Unit: the role of Severity Scoring Systems and general outcome prediction models (editorial). *Mayo Clin Proc* 2005;80(2):161–3.
7. Frick S, Uehlinger DE, Zuercher Zenklusen RM. Medical futility: predicting outcome of intensive care unit patients by nurses and doctors – a prospective comparative study. *Crit Care Med* 2003;31(2):456–61.
8. Kon AA, Shepard EK, Sederstrom NO, Swoboda SM, Marshall MF, Birriel B, et al. Defining futile and potentially inappropriate interventions: a policy statement from the Society of Critical Care Medicine Ethics Committee. *Crit Care Med* 2016;44(9):1769–74.

6

Withdrawing treatment

In their best interests

… and refusing to treat those who are overmastered by their diseases, realising that in such cases medicine is powerless.[1]

Hippocrates (450–380 BCE), Greek physician,
the 'Father of Medicine'

You don't treat me no good no more.

Sonia Dada, Blues band, in their song
You don't treat me no good (1992)

*

Withdrawing treatment in end-of-life care means stopping *life-sustaining* or *life support* treatment such as mechanical ventilation, infusions of drugs that stimulate the heart and sustain blood pressure and kidney dialysis. It is an agonising decision for patients, families and staff in end-of-life care. The withdrawal of treatment does not include withdrawing palliative care.

*

'They decided to withdraw treatment because it was futile. They did not need consent to do so, although they consulted your family. How did you feel about that?', I asked Mike my neighbour, when he was telling me about his grandmother's admission to hospital with a massive stoke.

'You know, it was weird', he said. 'We all thought we were given a black and white choice for Nana – *treatment and continuing with life* versus *no treatment and death*. Dad freaked out. He saw it as a decision on his Mum's life, you know, like making a moral judgment about the value of her life.' His eyes had a far-away look.

'It's more about making a decision in her best interests', I reassured him. 'Let me explain.'

*

History of withdrawing treatment

The act of withdrawing futile treatment goes a long way back in history. Hammurabi, the sixth king of Babylon,[a] enacted the Hammurabi code of law in about 1754 BCE, one of the world's oldest deciphered writings. It consists of 282 laws with rewards and punishments scaled according to social status: a free man or woman, or a slave. The code incorporated healthcare and specified that doctors merited esteem and rewards. While payment was good, punishments for severe and fatal errors were harsh, such as cutting off a surgeon's fingers and hands. This 'eye for an eye' justice affected medical practice in that doctors practised defensive medicine, abstaining or withdrawing from treating severe injuries or conditions likely to have a poor outcome. A legacy of the code's oppressive reprisals was regression of Babylonian medical progress.

Evidence of doctors' practices in ancient times is also disclosed in the Egyptian papyruses of Smith and Ebers. The *Smith papyrus*, written about 1700 BCE – the oldest known medical writing – is a treatise on surgery of antiquity. It describes almost 50 cases and recommends withdrawing treatment in 16 cases deemed incurable. The *Ebers papyrus*, dated to about 1552 BCE, is considered an ancient textbook on medicine and presents a case in which no treatment was advised.

---

[a] Babylon was a key kingdom in ancient Mesopotamia from the 18th to 6th centuries BCE. Mesopotamia was a historical region in West Asia situated within the Tigris–Euphrates river system, in modern days roughly corresponding to most of Iraq, Kuwait and parts of Saudi Arabia, Syria and Turkey.

Doctors over successive centuries accepted the practice of withdrawing futile interventions. This attitude was supported by philosophers such as Plato (437–347 BCE), who had an interest in defining the limits of medicine. Hippocrates (460–377 BCE) in ancient Greece left a legacy of three fundamental foundations of medicine: to free patients from suffering, to heal illness and to refrain from treating patients who are overcome with disease. In later centuries, medieval doctors adopted the Greek ideals on withdrawing futile treatment, but with a new scope of supplementing care of the terminally ill patient.

In Western medicine, the Christian tradition of philosophers and theologians contributed to ethical standards in medicine that included three fundamental elements: condemnation of suicide, preservation of life and possibility of withdrawing from excessively oppressive treatment. The writings of Francisco De Vitoria (1483–1546), a Spanish Dominican theologian, set the groundwork to develop the traditional teaching that distinguishes between 'ordinary' and 'extraordinary' means of preserving life. To prolong life in the face of imminent death, 'ordinary' means of treatment is required, but 'extraordinary' means that are burdensome to the patient may be discontinued. This moral obligatory view of the means of preserving life was a great achievement in the 16th century to offer moral solutions to withdrawing futile treatment.

*

Withdrawing and withholding treatment

Withdrawing or stopping *life support* treatment leads to poor oxygenation and heart function, or deranged body metabolism, which rapidly ends in death. *'To cure sometimes, to relieve often and to comfort always'* is an aphorism summarising the role of doctors. However, when treatment fails to cure and to preserve life, withdrawing or withholding such futile treatment is a fundamental component of end-of-life care. Withdrawing treatment does not mean stopping *all* treatment, but only life support interventions and unwarranted medications. The patient is by now unconscious, but pain relief, comfort measures and palliative medical and nursing care continue to be given.

Some media writers use the term 'passive euthanasia' to refer to withdrawal of treatment, painting it as killing by omission. This term is a poor choice because it can generate confusion and fear. Stopping futile life support treatment is not euthanasia (Chapter 10 Euthanasia) as the patient dies a death 'of natural causes' consequent to the illness.

By consensus, there is no legal or ethical difference between withdrawing treatment and withholding it. Some families and doctors view withdrawing treatment with a greater concern than withholding treatment. However, although the decision-making processes may differ, as withholding treatment is a prospective decision, the reasons that justify not introducing a treatment are the same ones that justify withdrawing it. Hence, treatments should not be withheld because of the mistaken fear that if begun, they cannot later be withdrawn. Instead, a time-limited trial of therapy could clarify the patient's prognosis, such as ventilation support for Jim Hockaday with motor neuron disease and mask-ventilation for Jason Black with end-stage respiratory failure.

Obviously, treatment is withheld or withdrawn when it is futile or inappropriate. The stage to withdraw or withhold treatment can vary, as predicting survival is not precise (Chapter 5 Prognostications). If death is anticipated to be quick, such as following withdrawal of mechanical ventilation, the intervention may be timed to allow family members to assemble.

Legal status of withdrawing or withholding treatment

The medical team can legally withdraw or withhold treatment if it is judged in the patient's 'best interests'. The principle of patient autonomy bestows the right to *refuse* treatment – a negative right to non-interference. By contrast, to interpret autonomy as a positive right – that is, a right to *demand* treatment – would arguably entitle everyone to *any* requested treatment, regardless of medical appropriateness or resources needed. This is often incompatible with practical realities and the ethical principles of non-maleficence (do no harm) and justice (fair use of resources). Hence, respect for patient autonomy need not overcome the patient's best interests in decisions to withdraw or withhold treatment. Respect for life does not mean that life must be preserved 'at all costs'.

The body of criminal law in Australia asserts that a person who voluntarily assumes responsibility for an incapacitated other has a duty to provide that incapacitated other with the 'necessaries of life'. In civil law, the law of negligence requires a doctor to use reasonable care and skill in making treatment decisions. However, in the few contested cases where families have sought to prevent their loved ones' treatment from being withdrawn or withheld by their attending doctors, the courts applied the standard of the patient's 'best interests'. The courts generally relied on doctors to determine futility. The cases of Messiha and Herrington are examples.

MESSIHA CASE

In 2004, a 75-year-old man presented to a New South Wales hospital's ICU after an out-of-hospital cardiac arrest with resultant severe hypoxic brain damage. He had chronic lung and heart disease and had suffered a previous cardiac arrest. There was no advance care directive. He remained in deep coma, and an independent neurologist confirmed his irrecoverable severe brain damage. The ICU doctors discussed withdrawing mechanical ventilation with the family, who disagreed and initiated court action to continue full treatment. The trial judge upheld the doctors' clinical decision, in the patient's best interests, on the evidence that treatment was futile without evidence of a resulting 'significant recovery' (of the brain).

HERRINGTON CASE

The Victorian Supreme Court declined to order that active treatment be continued for a woman with hypoxic brain damage who had been in a persistent vegetative state for six months. It held that 'there would be no clinical justification for the administration of any treatment, other than by way of palliative care'.

Determination of futility cannot be premature, as shown in the next case.

NORTHRIDGE CASE

The New South Wales Supreme Court reinstated active treatment for a 37-year-old man in a coma from a heroin overdose. It held that his doctors' diagnosis of 'chronic vegetative state' and their decision to withdraw treatment were premature, and thus not in Mr Northridge's best interests.

The objective standard of 'best interests' allows decisions independent of the patient's presumed personal values, and places more emphasis on futility than US courts. There is no duty to provide treatment that is futile, and medical professional bodies support this counsel.[b] The courts have also determined that 'overly burdensome' treatment, relative to benefits, is not in the patient's best interests. In assessing best-interests relevance, the courts have not considered the interests of other parties, including health authorities. Thus, costs of care have not been a major consideration in decisions to allow withdrawal of treatment, unlike decisions made in American courts.

Withdrawing treatment in overseas jurisdictions

In New Zealand, the duty to provide the necessaries of life is contained in the *Crimes Act 1961* (NZ). In two cases, the court determined 'good medical practice' in the patient's best interests as a 'lawful excuse' to breach this duty. In one, withdrawal of mechanical ventilation was judged lawful 'where there is no medical justification' to continue ventilation, although mechanical ventilation was accepted as a necessary of life. In the other, renal dialysis was withheld lawfully, in 'conformity with prevailing medical standards and with practices, procedures and traditions commanding general approval within the medical profession'. This position of 'good medical practice' to withdraw or withhold futile treatment as an excuse of the criminal code is untested in Australia.

In the UK the *Adults with Incapacity (Scotland) Act 2000* and the *Mental Capacity Act 2005* are laws on decision making for patients who lack capacity. The latter was enacted following the

---

[b]   e.g. the Medical Board of Australia's *Good medical practice: a code of conduct for doctors in Australia*[2]:

3.12.3 Understanding the limits of medicine in prolonging life and recognising when efforts to prolong life may not benefit the patient.

3.12.4 Understanding that you do not have a duty to try to prolong life at all cost. However, you do have a duty to know when not to initiate and when to cease attempts at prolonging life, while ensuring that your patients receive appropriate relief from distress.

Bland case, and a best-interests standard seems to be the test in English law.

BLAND CASE

In 1989, 17-year-old Anthony Bland became a victim of the Hillsborough disaster, a soccer ground in Sheffield, England, where 95 fans were crushed to death in the stadium's overcrowded stands. Although Bland survived the initial crush, he had suffered crushed ribs and punctured lungs, resulting in oxygen insufficiency and severe hypoxic brain damage. Months later, after no improvement in his persistent vegetative state, his doctors and his parents applied to court to withdraw his tube feeding. The Official Solicitor (who acts for children or the disabled) as his guardian *ad litem* opposed the application, arguing that withdrawing nutrition and hydration would be an active act to bring about death, which would amount to manslaughter or murder. The court supported the application, but the Official Solicitor appealed to the Court of Appeal. This was dismissed, as was a second appeal to the House of Lords in 1992. All judges at the three levels unanimously recognised that it is lawful to withdraw artificial feeding from a patient in a persistent vegetative state. The courts decreed nutrition and hydration as a medical treatment, and characterised its cessation as an omission and not an act, and therefore not regarded as criminal conduct. As there was no prospect of treatment improving his vegetative state, they judged treatment as futile. There was hence no duty to continue nutrition and hydration because that was not in his best interests.

Bland never regained consciousness, and died on 3 March 1993, aged 22, after being in a coma for nearly four years. Thus, hydration and nutrition are regarded as a life-sustaining treatment that can lawfully be withdrawn or withheld from a dying patient who lacks capacity, if the treatment is not in their best interests. However, to do so from a patient in a persistent vegetative state or similar condition such as Bland, the laws in England, Wales and Northern Ireland still require a court ruling.[3]

In America, courts have considered autonomy, best interests, *substituted judgment* (deducing what the patient would have wanted) and the sanctity of life, in cases of withdrawing and withholding treatment in patients without capacity. A number of legal cases in the 1970s and 1980s provided the impetus to develop laws relevant to withdrawing or withholding life-sustaining treatments, beginning with the *Quinlan* case, which attracted worldwide publicity.

QUINLAN CASE

In 1975, Karen Quinlan, a 22-year-old woman, became unconscious at a party in New Jersey. The cause was never established, but she had apparently consumed alcohol and tranquillisers. She showed signs of severe hypoxic brain damage and, after weeks on a ventilator in ICU, was in a persistent vegetative state. Karen's father petitioned a trial court to be named her guardian so that he could direct ventilation to be stopped. Her doctors were opposed, and they maintained that she was medically and legally alive, although dependent on the ventilator to breathe. They did not want to violate the prevailing medical standards and practices. The trial judge agreed with the doctors, reasoning that what Mr Quinlan sought would allow his daughter to die, which was 'not something in her best interests'. Mr Quinlan then appealed to the New Jersey Supreme Court, which overturned the decision of the lower court, appointing Mr Quinlan as Karen's guardian. The state Supreme Court ruled that if Karen were competent, she would have a 'constitutional right of privacy' to decide against further mechanical ventilation. Ventilation was 'extraordinary care' for irreversibly unconscious patients, which the state could not compel her to endure 'with no realistic possibility of returning to any semblance of a cognitive or sapient life'. Her 'constitutional right of privacy' overcame the state's interest in preserving life. As she could not exercise this right on her own, her father acting as her guardian could exert it. Karen's ventilator was then discontinued but, unexpectedly, she was able to breathe on her own. She survived for another nine years in a nursing home and never regained consciousness.

Present-day ICU doctors will wonder why Karen Quinlan's doctors did not initially wean her off the ventilator, as she was not brain dead and therefore able to breathe on her own (Chapter 9 Brain death and vegetative states). Perhaps they misunderstood the concepts of brain death, which was defined at that time in the US by the 1968 *Ad Hoc Committee of the Harvard Medical School to Examine the Definition of Brain Death*. Her father had not sought other medical care to be stopped, apparently because he had moral problems with depriving his daughter of nutrition and antibiotics. Nonetheless, in the wake of this case, most US states confirmed the right of competent patients to refuse treatment and of surrogate decision making for incapacitated patients.

CRUZAN CASE

The *Cruzan* case tested the issue of withdrawing a feeding tube that provided nutrition and hydration. Nancy Cruzan, a 25-year-old woman, overturned her car in 1983, landed face-down in a ditch and suffered severe hypoxic brain damage. After weeks in a coma, she was confirmed to be in a persistent vegetative state. She required only tube feeding, with no ventilator support to stay alive in a Missouri hospital. After four years with no improvement, her parents applied to court to have her feeding tube removed and allow her to die a 'dignified death' as, according to them, she would have wanted. The trial judge decided in their favour, but the State of Missouri, supported by a coalition of right-to-life advocates, fought them all the way to the US Supreme Court. This high court decided against the Cruzans. It upheld the legal standard that incapacitated persons or their surrogates have the right to refuse medical treatment, but recognised the state's interest in preserving life and its right to establish parameters before such decisions can be made. As Nancy was unable to exercise her right, the State of Missouri required a 'clear and convincing evidence' of her rejection of her treatment. In response, her parents provided more proof that she would not have wanted her life-sustaining treatments, and finally won a court order in 1990 to have her tube feeding stopped. She died 11 days later, after almost eight years in coma with rigid limbs, occasional seizures and no cognition ability. In setting the high legal standard of evidence required, the courts held that the sanctity of life remains absolute. This case differs from *Quinlan* in its withdrawal of nutrition and hydration instead of ventilation, and that death ensued shortly afterwards, but, like *Quinlan*, the courts did not primarily address the concept of futility.

Although advance care directives or 'living wills' had been available for some years, following this widely publicised case the US Congress in 1990 passed the *Patient Self-Determination Act* to promote ACDs on a national level. A decade later, the *Schiavo* case was another high-profile, complex legal saga, but extraordinary in its interference by third parties and politicians.

SCHIAVO CASE

In 1990, 26-year-old Terri Schiavo mysteriously collapsed at home and suffered severe hypoxic brain damage. For the next few years, her husband Michael Schiavo and her parents, the Schindlers, worked together in efforts to rehabilitate her. She remained unresponsive in a persistent vegetative state, requiring feeding through a gastrostomy (a tube surgically inserted from the abdomen to the stomach). Her husband then insisted that she would not want to live this way, and petitioned the Florida guardianship court to review her life-prolonging procedures. Her parents resisted any move to withdraw treatment. In 2000, the trial court decided that she met the statutory definition of persistent vegetative state, with no hope of regaining consciousness. The court then found 'clear and convincing evidence' of Terri's wishes, from witnesses' statements of her past oral announcements that 'she would not want to live like that', and ordered the feeding tube to be removed. The Schindlers appealed, starting a seven-year legal battle that went all the way to the US Supreme Court. They held that their daughter's unconscious state was not permanent, and that she would have wanted to live. In one appellate hearing, the Schindlers presented affidavits from a radiologist and a neurologist – *who had not examined Terri* – that she was not in a persistent vegetative state, and that she could be helped by certain medical treatment. That appeal was lost when independent, court-appointed neurologists all affirmed Terri's irreversible brain damage as persistent vegetative state. The court also found the Schindlers' experts' evidence and their rehabilitation theories unconvincing, and once again ordered the withdrawal of the feeding tube in October 2003. Jeb Bush, Florida's Governor, overruled this a few days later, when he signed 'Terri's Law' to order resumption of her tube feeding. The Florida Supreme Court then found Bush's law unconstitutional, and the feeding tube was removed in March 2005, despite an attempt by President George W. Bush to override the Florida courts. Terri Schiavo died on 31 March 2005, ending 14 court appeals and numerous hearings and petitions, protests by pro-life and disability rights groups and interference by the Florida Governor and the US President. An autopsy showed extensive, hypoxic brain damage.

Using a *human rights* concept to oppose withdrawing or withholding life-sustaining treatment has not been contested in courts in Australia. In the UK in 2005, a 45-year-old Mr Leslie Burke, with a degenerative brain condition, challenged in court the General Medical Council's (GMC's) guide[4] in giving doctors the ultimate say on what treatment to give a patient like him in the final stages, arguing that it was an infringement of his human rights.[5] His case lost on appeal, but the GMC reassured him that nothing in its guidance prevented his receiving the treatment he would need.

*

Mike leaned back in his chair, nursing his beer with both hands in silent contemplation of what I had told him. 'Very interesting', he said finally. 'But what does "best interests" mean? Surely it's subjective, pure speculation?'

'That's true in part', I said. 'Like "futility", there's no consensus of a definition of "best interests". Its consideration first evaluates benefits of continuing care – in your grandma the probability of survival is almost nil – versus liabilities of continuing futile treatment, what we call "burdensome care". These include discomfort, pain, suffering, compromise of dignity and loss of cognition – everything intolerable. Then the doctors, nurses and your family discuss her wishes and feelings, past and present, including religious or moral beliefs based on views she had previously expressed, as well as any insight your dad or family and friends can offer. In a nutshell, it's end-of-life care encompassing medical, physical, emotional and all other factors relevant to your grandma's welfare. It's meant to be a shared decision, but the doctors can have the final say.'

Mike took a sip of his beer, his forehead wrinkled in doubt. 'Don't know about that. They didn't ask Dad to sign a formal consent to stop treatment.'

*

Family discussions and consent

In discussing withdrawing treatment, the patient's family, like my neighbour's, may see themselves presented with a simple choice of two options: 'no' to continue treatment, or 'yes' to withdraw.

When framed in this manner, the 'yes' choice has connotations of 'giving up' or 'cutting our losses', a negative option that implies abandoning hope, which can appear to families as really no option at all. Ethnic sensitivities with cultural and religious beliefs of doctors, patients and families may also influence attitudes to withdraw treatment (Chapter 12 Religions at the end of life, Chapter 13 Cultures and ethnicities).

Doctors have no duty to provide treatment deemed to be futile, and in the absence of such a duty to treat they may then unilaterally withdraw or withhold treatment. In withholding treatment, doctors may withhold information about interventions judged too futile to offer. Obligations to secure consent to withhold such treatment are not powerful. However, in withdrawing futile treatment, the doctors should consult with the family. The aim of discussions with the family is to inform, and to share decision making to individualise end-of-life care. However, the role of consent, including the imperative to secure informed consent, is less clear. In practice, consent to withdraw or withhold treatment is generally seen as not mandated. Of the Australian states' and territories' guardianship or medical consent legislations, it is likely that only Queensland's requires consent to withdraw or withhold such futile treatment.[6] The situation in New Zealand is uncertain.

In the UK, the legal principles around consent are the same for all medical interventions, including decisions to withdraw or withhold life-sustaining treatment. Where an incapacitated adult has no one to make a decision on their behalf, treatment can be provided in the patient's best interests. Professional guidelines give a high priority to discussions with the patient's family, but the legal status of their decisions or consent to withdraw or withhold treatment in adults is unclear. Withdrawing nutrition and hydration from patients in a persistent vegetative state, as previously stated, requires a court referral.

In the US, withdrawing and withholding life support is legally justified primarily by the principles of informed consent and informed refusal, both of which have strong roots in the common law. Statutory and case law vary from state to state, but limiting life-sustaining treatment is legally justified only if it represents unwanted treatment and *has the consent* of patients or their surrogates. Doctors may base their recommendations on futility, but this concept should not be invoked to remove life support without the knowledge of patients or their substitute decision makers, or over their objections. For incompetent patients who lack a substitute decision maker, doctors or the hospital's ethics body, if there is one, may decide in the patients' best interests.

*

Rosemary Smith stuck her head in my office. 'You need to come quick!', she said with a harried grimace. 'Angelo DiMasso is causing a ruckus in the waiting room.' Angelo was the 19-year-old youngest son of Vince, the elderly patient in bed 12. The patriarch of the DiMasso family had been admitted three weeks previously with severe abdominal and chest injuries, the result of a farm accident. Vince's condition had deteriorated owing to sepsis and he was now in multiorgan failure. An hour ago I had informed his wife, four sons and a large group of relatives that his prognosis was grim. Withdrawing treatment could be a consideration if his condition deteriorated further and care became futile.

The waiting room is a large room at the entry into ICU, adjacent to the reception desk. The four seated adults in the room, relatives of other patients, looked alarmed. Their source of discomfort was Angelo, standing at the doorway, addressing his large family group of 14, all standing, clustered inside and outside the room. He was distressed and agitated, gesticulating and waving his arms, bawling words and tears. 'They want to stop Papa's treatment! They want to do euthanasia! They want to kill him!', he sobbed, with his mother crying softly beside him. Two hospital security guards arrived but I waved them away. We somehow managed to calm and comfort Angelo and his mother, and the family eventually shepherded them outside the ICU.

I always make three points clear to families. First, if the life-sustaining treatment is judged to be futile, discontinuing burdensome treatment is in their loved one's best interests. Secondly, withdrawing futile treatment does not mean abandoning care. Finally, withdrawing treatment is not euthanasia. The act of omission is not to end life, but rather to discontinue futile treatment so as not to delay inevitable death.

Mike's grandmother did not make an ACD. She died pain free (so far as we know) in the presence of her family. It might not have been how she would have chosen to die, as Mike alluded to.

*

Reflections

- There is no difference ethically and legally between withdrawing treatment and withholding treatment that is futile and burdensome to the patient.
- Withdrawing treatment does not mean withdrawing all care, especially palliative care.
- Doctors should discuss withdrawing futile treatment with the family, without needing formal informed consent.
- Families should understand why treatment is judged futile, what the options of care (if any) are, what specific treatments will be withdrawn and what will not, and the timeframe of withdrawing life-sustaining treatments.
- The healthcare team should advise and help the family attend to their relative's important matters before death, e.g. a life insurance policy. Counselling support should be arranged if needed for families and staff.

References

1. Jones WHS, editor. *Hippocrates II*. Cambridge MA: Harvard University Press; 1923. p. 193.
2. Medical Board of Australia. *Good medical practice: a code of conduct for doctors in Australia*. Barton, ACT: AHPRA; 2014. https://www.medicalboard.gov.au/Codes-Guidelines-Policies/Code-of-conduct.aspx.
3. General Medical Council. *Treatment and care towards the end of life: good practice in decision making*. London: GMC; 2010.
4. General Medical Council. *Withholding and withdrawing life-prolonging treatments*. London: GMC; 2002.
5. United Nations. *Universal Declaration of Human Rights, Article 3, The right to life, liberty and security of a person*. Geneva: UN; 1948. www.un.org/en/universal-declaration-human-rights.
6. Willmott L, White B, Downie J. Withholding and withdrawal of 'futile' life-sustaining treatment: unilateral medical decision-making in Australia and New Zealand. *J Law Med* 2013;20:907.

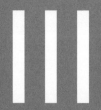

PART

Communication

Communication

We need to talk about Kevin[a]

The single biggest problem in communication is the illusion that it has taken place.

George Bernard Shaw (1856–1950),
Irish playwright, Nobel Laureate

The two words information and communication are often used interchangeably, but they signify quite different things. Information is giving out; communication is getting through.

Sydney Harris (1917–86), Chicago journalist

*

Effective communication is an essential skill for health professionals. Good communication is critical in managing patients with serious illness and their families to provide information, counsel and comfort, and to listen effectively to their wishes and concerns. There is no better example than family conversations in end-of-life care.

*

---

[a] Novel by Lionel Shriver[1] and film directed by Lynne Ramsay 2011.

It was the weekly lunch-hour hospital 'grand round', when an invited speaker delivers a talk of interest to the hospital's doctors, nurses and allied health staff. The speaker this week was Dr Gaylene Bennett, a psychologist and human relations consultant based at the health department head office, or the 'Kremlin' as known by staff.

She was finishing her talk after 40 minutes, '... patient-centred care has moral implications with deep respect for patients as unique clients in context of their own social worlds. Use the term in your communication lexicon to vocalise its essential and revolutionary meaning: to diminish the drudgery of productivity-driven, assembly-line medicine and cognitive overload. Doctors and nurses should invite your clients to participate in meaningful holistic deliberations of shared minds.'

The audience had started to trickle out of the lecture theatre halfway thorough her talk, but that cascaded into a stampede when she finished. There were no questions from the stalwarts who remained. No one had understood much of what she had actually said, although her topic, 'Communication in healthcare', was ironically clear.

Dr Bennett's talk reminded me of my bicycle ride the preceding Sunday morning. 'It's fuck-a-brass-monkey-duck cold', exclaimed Anton Jelinek, a member of our peloton who had emigrated to Australia 6 months before. English not being his first language, from time to time he offered interesting metaphors. He was right though. It was brass-monkey cold at 5.30 a.m. that morning. He had communicated that fact to our group passionately and clearly, in contrast to the murkiness of Dr Bennett's talk.

What is communication?

Communication is a key element of living, especially of relationships, and communication skills are important qualities in business and professional practices. In medicine, this means doctors exchanging information on medical care with patients, families, nurses and colleagues. Basic reading, writing and listening skills learned at school and university, although important, are not enough for doctors to communicate effectively, which can then affect patient outcome.

Communication can be verbal or written. Varied techniques and skills are necessary for doctors to communicate. In clinical emergencies, lead doctors need to direct nurses and colleagues with clear, unambiguous, single-task instructions targeted at individuals. Good communication between interdisciplinary colleagues will minimise disagreements among staff and enhance quality of care and patient safety. A crucial component is handing over clinical information, such as when the patient is transferred from one team to another. Poor handovers raise risks of medical mishaps (Chapter 17 Medical mishaps). The rest of this chapter looks at communication between doctors and patients and families. Two issues are relevant in ICU. Many patients are unconscious or sedated, and may sometimes recall events when awake, with possible psychological outcomes. ICU doctors and nurses need to regard them, and verbally address them, as if they were awake, especially when performing procedures on them. Secondly, doctors frequently communicate with families, as many patients are incapacitated.

Doctors today practise evidence-based medicine and *'patient-centred care'*. The latter, in contrast to *'disease-orientated care'*, provides care that respects individual patient preferences and values. Hence effective communication preserves a successful doctor–patient relationship. For incapacitated patients, family members are substitute decision makers. Doctors then speak with the family, and the attributes of effective communication still apply, but there are nuances (see later in this chapter). Good communicating skills help the doctor to *seek* information in history taking, *explain* the diagnosis and illness, *provide* counselling and *discuss* and *share* decisions on treatment. There are potential physical and emotional benefits to the patient and the family, who are more likely to comply with treatment. Better mental health and tolerance of pain in patients have been reported. Family satisfaction is another consequence of good communication. Complaints by patients' families about hospital doctors are fortunately uncommon in Australia, but most of them are about poor communication: their doctors had provided inadequate information, had not bothered to *really* listen to them and their concerns were not allayed or addressed. They felt excluded from decision making and cheated by the inadequate time the doctors had given them.

Finally, good communication improves patient safety. Poor doctor–nurse communication errors in the ICU are associated with medical mishaps (Chapter 17 Medical mishaps).[2] Good collaborative communication can result in improved patient mortality rates and shorter hospital stays. All these factors influence the choices that patients and families make, which may then significantly affect care. Indeed, communication may be the most important factor in end-of-life care, such as in discussions on withdrawing treatment. Families who experienced good communication approaches reported less anxiety and depression with better perceptions of quality of death of their relatives.[3]

*

'You know, in that two days nana was in the ICU, there must've been 20 different doctors who spoke to mum and dad about her care. We knew that she had suffered a stroke and that it was massive, but we didn't fully understand what we were told, and how or why they decided that the prognosis was hopeless. Medical terms – jingoistic jargon – were spewed like the trots. One young neurologist, arrogant prick, kept looking at his watch. Confused us no end. Contradicted what the ICU docs had told us an hour before. Said he was from Melbourne; they must speak a different lingo there … I'm in advertising, Tom. These guys couldn't talk a root out of a penniless hooker. Are you guys always so tongue-twisted? We got more lucid information from the ICU cleaner!' Mike, my neighbour, threw up his hands, his eyes wide in frustration. He was describing his family's experience with the way doctors had communicated with them about his grandmother. Indeed, he communicated clearly to me that he was unimpressed.

*

Doctors communicate poorly

With the evolution from paternalistic to patient-centred care, not all doctors have successfully negotiated the change with respect to communication skills. Some may overestimate their abilities when their perception of adequate communication is not supported by discontent expressed by their patients.

Why are there problems in doctors communicating with patients or families? Traditionally, many doctors consider it brutal and harmful to patients to disclose the full gamut of bad news because of bleak prognoses. Doctors are also wary that they might not have the time or capacity to cope with the consequential social and emotional distress that bad news can evoke. Some struggle with a difficult family discussion, simply viewing it as a chore, with attending conflicts just chalking up their job stress. Acute care doctors of incapacitated patients often face families who are distressed and distraught, and some family members with strong emotions can be demanding and even abrasive. The doctors may stonewall such attitudes, even though stress provoked, with a view of '*them taking it out on us.*'

*

'We freaked out the first time we entered the ICU. You get overwhelmed by the sight of machines and monitors and lights and alarms. Patients with tubes coming from all orifices, all lined up in beds like open coffins, one step away from death. All are *incommunicado*, attached to wires and drips and ventilators and monitors. It's a shit-scaring environment the first time, if you have family in one of those beds', John my weekly cycling mate said. We were having coffee at our favourite pit-stop café after our Sunday morning ride. He was recounting his experience when his uncle was admitted to the ICU after major bowel cancer surgery. 'Thank God I didn't have to go in repeatedly every day, like aunt Norma and my cousins.'

*

Factors affecting how families communicate

A number of factors resulting from a relative being seriously ill in hospital may affect how families receive bad news and handle decision making. The hospital environment, particularly acute care areas like the emergency department, operating theatres and ICU, can be daunting to patients and families, and can adversely influence family experiences. Family members may be in a state of 'fear and shock' initially when they see that their relative is dependent on machines and drugs to remain alive, *and yet may still die*. In that unsettling environment, their burden of coping with their potential loss is increased by many factors: the expectation to be the patient's advocate, financial problems from hospital costs and disruption of home and job routines. The considerable time spent at the bedside, directing their energies to the patient while neglecting their own needs, and the exhausting grind of making multiple daily trips to the hospital, take a toll on the physical health of some members. Existing or resultant underlying tensions between family members may become even more strained. Consequently, many families report psychological symptoms from their experience; anxiety, traumatic stress and depression are common, especially if the patient's illness and recovery are prolonged.[4] Indeed, some family members may even experience feelings of disorganisation and symptoms of posttraumatic stress disorder (PTSD) 3–12 months after the death of their relative.[5] The psychosocial impact that a patient's hospital admission has on family members can result in strong emotions in some family members. All these issues may affect how families respond in communicating with doctors.

*

'What a weirdo', Alicia said in the staff room during her break. She was the nurse of Mrs Jane Cordingley in bed 13, who had been admitted in a coma two days previously. She had collapsed when moving a heavy pot plant, and CT scans showed a ruptured cerebral aneurysm. It was a massive vascular stroke that was inoperable, and her deteriorating clinical status reflected her poor prognosis. 'He kissed her on the cheek, sat down and proceeded to tell me jokes', she said, eyebrows raised in sympathy and puzzlement. She was referring to Jim Cordingley, the husband. 'He behaved is if he was at a morning tea party', she continued. 'Does he not understand that she will die soon?' she said, looking at me as she jiggled her tea bag in her mug.

I knew what she meant. His demeanour when I talked with him in the interview room on the day of her admission was not that of an overwrought spouse. Indeed it was weird. Well-dressed, tie-less in a white shirt and smart grey suit, he did not appear concerned or worried, and, although he fidgeted in his seat, he seemed as keen and almost jovial as a boy scout. 'Jane's prognosis is extremely poor', I had told him. 'You understand, don't you, that her stroke is massive, beyond life-saving surgery? I'm sorry but she is highly likely to die', I concluded to ensure that he did not miss my message.

'Thank you doc', he had replied. His face was expressionless. He then shrugged his shoulders with a wry smile. 'We all have to go sometime.'

I was about to reply to Alicia when Felicity spoke. 'Give me Mr Cordingley any day. You can have Mr Gorky. That man's arrogant, crass, rude and abusive. He told me that we are lucky that his son hadn't died because of our poor nursing care – and all doctors are greedy incompetents.'

Vladimir Gorky was the father of 17-year-old Alex Gorky in bed 8. The young Gorky had wrapped his car around a tree when speeding while drunk. He suffered fractured ribs and pelvis and underwent emergency surgery to remove his ruptured spleen. The elder Gorky, a former teenage immigrant, had worked hard to become a wealthy used-car yard owner. He was angry with his son but seemed more so with everyone else, having made three complaints to the hospital about the 'shonky' treatment that his son was receiving. Clearly, he compared the healthcare profession to his used-car business.

*

EMOTIONS AFFECTING HOW FAMILIES COMMUNICATE

Family members of critically ill ICU patients may develop strong emotions and incongruous behaviour, which are not conducive to the patient's care or the emotional needs of the family, but are a normal psychosocial response to trauma, anxiety and uncertainty. Inappropriate emotions and behavioural responses may be expressed as anger, hostility, truculence and also ineffective communication. On a positive note, families with stable interpersonal relations are good communicators and a valuable source of emotional support for the patient. Doctors and nurses must be cognisant with these factors as well as those associated with culture (Chapter 13 Cultures and ethnicities) and religion (Chapter 12 Religions at the end of life) in communicating with families.

Emotions are fundamental to human experience and behaviour. An emotional reaction is a physical response to a 'trigger' (such as a situation, event or dialogue), which activates the limbic system in the brain. Released neurotransmitters instigate biochemical reactions that alter physical states in the body. Varying patterns of brain activation give rise to different emotions, the basic emotions being *happiness*, *sadness*, *anger*, *fear*, *surprise* and *disgust*. Emotions, being physical states, can be objectively measured by blood flow, brain activity, facial microexpressions and body language.

Feelings are different. A 'feeling' is a sensation experienced via touch, smell, sight or any other sensory organ, but feelings can also originate in the higher-order (neocortical) regions of the brain. These feelings are mental associations and reactions to emotions, and arise when the brain perceives and assigns meanings to emotions (although feelings can also trigger emotions). Feelings are subjective, involving cognitive input (usually sub-conscious), and are influenced by personal experience, beliefs and memories. As feelings are mental experiences, they cannot be measured precisely. For example, when confronted by a snarling dog, the body responds to this external trigger event, and we experience the *emotion of fear*, reflected physically as sweating, trembling, etc. and mentally as a *feeling of terror*.

Emotions of distressed family members of patients are triggered by the event of their loved one's illness, and perhaps from care that they might consider suboptimal. Other triggers of emotions are a sense of helplessness, and the lack of attention, respect and fair treatment that they think they are accorded, but are less than what they believe they deserve. In the hospital context, the same scenario may evoke different emotions in different people, especially those of different cultures. Expressions of emotional response of family members can include sorrow, fatigue, depression, relief, shock, guilt, frustration and anxiety.[6] Almost every emotion and their accompanying behaviour can be considered as a normal response to the prospect of death and grief, as long as the behaviour is not self-destructive or illegal. Anger, as exhibited by Vladimir Gorky, is a common emotion, often a reaction to frustration or sometimes guilt. He had allowed his son to use his Mercedes to attend a 21st birthday party where alcohol would be abundant. The individual may project his anger onto the patient, a family member or the healthcare staff. Indifference, lack of concern, or even frivolity, as exhibited by Jim Cordingley towards his dying wife, are uncommon, but this conduct can be a coping mechanism – that of denial – allowing him to limit his consciousness about the reality of the inevitable death of his spouse.[7] Indeed, humour has been proposed as a counselling therapy for grief.[8] Denial can range from slight distortions of reality to full-blown delusions. Jim Cordingley had administered 'emotional anaesthesia' to himself, but when his wife died he wept openly, his need for denial gone.

Depending on gender roles, culture and situation, genders may differ in how much emotion they express. In developed Western countries, women appear to display more emotion than men, but men tend to express anger more, particularly towards strangers. Women may experience stronger negative emotions, which may be associated with their being more open in expressing feelings. The basic emotions are universal to all cultures whereas other aspects differ across cultures. Different cultures may categorise emotions differently, and some languages have words for emotions that are non-existent in other languages. The same situation or trigger event may evoke different emotional responses in different cultures. Prioritisation of emotions may also be different. For example, in Asian countries, shame is considered a key primary emotion. Apart from speech, emotions can also be expressed through non-verbal behaviour or body language. These include facial expressions, postures and gestures. To add to the complexity of cultural differences, non-verbal expressions of emotion differ across cultures, partly because of different etiquettes of behaviour. For example, many Asians tend not to display emotions despite feelings of sadness and grief. Physiological indicators of emotion are, however, similar in people of all cultures.

For families grappling to understand their relative's illness and varied treatment scenarios, their emotions may influence cognition, particularly attention, memory and decision making.[9] Intuition suggests that strong emotions may adversely affect reasoning. Indeed, 'happy' emotion-related processes can sometimes help reasoning and judgment in certain research scenarios, perhaps because of emotions enhancing perceptual abilities. Be that as it may, there is yet no conclusive evidence of how emotions affect decision making, but this issue is a consideration in communicating with families under risk and uncertainty.

*

Mr Wilhelm was a big, handsome, middle-aged man, almost two metres in height. He looked distinguished, dressed immaculately in a white silk shirt, black double-breasted suit and a red tie. 'John Wilhelm', he said, 'I'm the brother of Carol Cornelius.' He extended his hand with a courteous smile. 'Tell me about my sister.'

We were in the interview room, just the two of us. Carol Cornelius was a 60-year-old who had undergone elective anterior resection surgery that morning for colon cancer. Admission to ICU was a routine procedure following her major surgery to stabilise her physiological and biochemical responses and to provide optimal pain management.

'I have spoken with the surgeon, Dr Benson', John Wilhelm said. He folded his arms, exuding polite authority. 'He explained why he performed open laparotomy rather than laparoscopic key-hole surgery.' John Wilhelm was obviously a man who did not waste time. 'How is she doing now?' I informed him in some detail of the care we were giving her, and that her vital signs were stable.

He asked a few incisive questions about blood transfusion and pain relief measures. 'You know she's on heart and blood pressure medications', he said. 'According to her GP, these should continue without omission.' He expected an intelligent answer.

'Yes. I have prescribed them to be given intravenously.'

'If there is anything wrong or that you're concerned about, you must ring Dr Benson *and me*. Any time of day and night. You have my phone number?'

'Of course', I assured him. 'That's our usual procedure.'

'If she needs extra special care, I shall move her to St Mary's.'

'There is no need. This is a tertiary teaching hospital. We have all facilities, more than many private hospitals', I assured him.

He fixed his eyes at mine, looking unconvinced. He was not used to being contradicted. 'When will you discharge her back to her ward?'

'If she continues to remain stable, as I expect, she will be moved back to ward 7 tomorrow morning, after our ward round', I answered.

He sat up in his chair and unfolded his arms. 'I would not want her to be moved until she is perfectly ready to do so, and only if a private room is available. Indeed, it would be good if she remains here for at least another day', he said calmly. He looked sternly at me, firm in what he wanted and expecting his directives to be followed.

*

Communication skills

We teach communication skills to junior colleagues and medical students. To start with, the needs of families in discussions with doctors are identified as:

- to have questions answered honestly
- to feel that the staff care about the patient
- to know details about the patient's progress, and
- to know the expected outcome.[10]

The need for reassurance is as important as the need for information. Stage actors, when they first make their entrance, 'feel the room' – meaning that they *suss out* the audience to gain an ambience of their mood, responsiveness and appreciation. This tip applies when the doctor makes initial contact with family members in the interview room, trying to sense attitudes, personalities and emotional lability that may help flag potential obstacles. The family conversation can proceed along different communication styles. John Wilhelm, as I found out later, was a director of a large mining company. He seemed to view conversations with doctors like a board meeting, where junior executives (the doctors) report developments, whence he would give directions to proceed. His *family autonomy style* where the doctor merely provides information is at the opposite end of the family conversation spectrum to that of the *paternalism style*. Clearly, a halfway *collaborative* or *facilitative style* is the best form of communication, where the doctor informs and recommends, and the family asks and discusses. With this approach, the family conversation has three parts: setup, content and skill set.

Setup starts with a staff pre-meeting in which it is decided what to achieve at the meeting, who should speak and what to say. Everyone is briefed on the names of key family members, family dynamics, religious and cultural overlays and any issues of guilt or anger, and, if so, the reasons why. Team members should be cognisant of the patient's latest clinical status, and of the family's expectations that staff are respectful of their values and demonstrate sensitivity, empathy, honesty, sincerity, diligence and competence.

The meeting is scheduled at a time convenient to the family in a room conducive to private conversations, such as a dedicated interview room, and never at the bedside or in an ad hoc location like a corridor. Adequate time is scheduled and that time must be free of interruptions. Families expect their doctors to be appropriately dressed; anything too leisurely can be jarring.

Content starts with the lead doctor introducing the staff members *and their roles*, and asking the family members what they already know about the patient's condition. This is important to determine misconceptions or incorrect information that was previously given. Staff members then provide details of the patient's condition, treatment and prognosis, and make recommendations for treatment choices, giving reasons why. The family is informed of their loved one's pain relief measures – a top concern of families – and that of available support mechanisms, an important family need. If the prognosis is bleak, the lead doctor explains end-of-life care. The conversation is more about goals than about specific treatments. Staff and family ascertain the patient's values, such as wishes if an advanced care directive exists. Should the directive or the family's wish be inappropriate or illegal, this is explained to the family. If end-of-life care includes withdrawing life support treatment, central points are clarified: further continuing treatment is futile, burdensome to the patient and only delays inevitable death (Chapter 6 Withdrawing treatment). A decision to withdraw the futile treatment is ethical and legal, will not increase suffering and is compatible with the patient's values. If a patient is considered a potential organ donor, the organ donation specialist is involved. The specialist explains to the family that, in considering their consent, they have an opportunity to save a transplant recipient's life (Chapter 11 Organ donation).

Skill set is the skills of communication reflecting insight, observation, sensitivity, empathy, understanding and discernment (*see Box*). Eye contact, body language and appropriate touch can help convey warmth and empathy. Families want their doctors to know how they feel and what they want. For doctors to communicate effectively, skills need to be taught and be bolstered by feedback from superiors and peers. Such vital skills do not reliably improve with experience alone. With ageing, unlike a good wine, there is no guarantee of mellowed quality – no wisdom in talking. For this reason, specialist medical organisations such as the College of Intensive Care Medicine of Australia and New Zealand,[11] and DonateLife, Australia's organ donation body, incorporate mandatory courses in communication skills for their trainees and staff.

Communication Skill Set

- Conduct your conversation in 'tell/listen/ask' cycles.
- Speak clearly, using plain language and no jargon or unnecessary medical terms.
- Provide information in easy-to-follow 'chunks'.
- Repeat important points, pausing occasionally and checking the family's understanding – *'Does this make sense?'* or *'Shall I go over it again?'*
- Seek their impression of the illness. How close are their ideas to reality? What are their views of your care?
- Address their concerns.
- Elicit any issues of family conflict, culture, race, religion and social background.
- In breaking bad news, a 'warning shot' may be helpful – *'I'm afraid I've got bad news.'*
- Do not use euphemisms to 'soften the blow' as that may lead to vagueness and confusion.
- Listen actively and attentively, and never be paternalistic and patronising.
- Answer questions honestly. If you don't know the answer, promise to find out.
- Give the family time to digest and react to your information.
- It's a two-way information exchange. As the doctor, you need to know what are the patient's values and what does the family want for the patient?
- Always express support and record details of the meeting.

Finally, if the patient dies, grief can generate a range of emotions and feelings in the family that may be reflected in inappropriate, uncooperative or unconventional behaviour. Grief is a normal but complex response to loss (bereavement being the state of the loss) with varied expressions of emotions. There may be cognitive responses initially, such as disbelief, confusion and preoccupation with the loss of the deceased. In communicating with families, doctors should be cognisant of grief manifestations. Angry and hostile relatives dent our focus and job satisfaction. However, families need to be given support such as grief counselling, and managed with patience, empathy and assurance that good care accompanied their loved one's last journey.

*

I saw Rosemary Smith as I walked into the Department. 'Nursing admin rang me while you were away', she said. 'They received a complaint from the Brown family. No one told them about the time of Joe Brown's surgery. They missed greeting him when he came out of theatre. Also, Mr and Mrs Atkins came in bringing two big food hampers for the staff. Their son Alex is back at school and doing well. They expressed their gratitude for saving his life … and "honest information", their own words', she said with a smile. *One 'F' and one 'A' in communication*, I thought.

*

Reflections

- In communicating with patients and families, doctors should 'tell, listen and ask', and explain again any points that are unclear.
- All parties should be aware of other options for care.
- Any element of care that families are dissatisfied with should be addressed.
- Time allocated to the family discussion must be adequate; otherwise the doctor should arrange another meeting.
- Rudeness from any party is unacceptable.

References

1. Shriver L. *We need to talk about Kevin*. Berkeley, CA: Counterpoint; 2003.
2. Reader T, Flin R, Cuthbertson BH. Communications skills and error in the intensive care unit. *Curr Opin Crit Care* 2007;13(6):732–6.
3. Lautrette A, Darmon M, Megarbane B, Joly LM, Chevret S, Adrie C, et al. A communication strategy and brochure for relatives of patients dying in the ICU. *N Engl J Med* 2007;356(5):469–78.
4. McAdam JL, Fontaine DK, White DB, Dracup KA, Puntillo KA. Psychological symptoms of family members of high-risk intensive care unit patients. *Am J Crit Care* 2012;21(6):386–94.
5. Gries CJ, Engelberg RA, Kross EK, Zatzick D, Nielsen EL, Downey L, et al. Predictors of symptoms of posttraumatic stress and depression in family members after patient death in the ICU. *Chest* 2010;137(2):280–7.
6. Barbato A, Irwin H. Major therapeutic systems and the bereaved client. *Aust Psychol* 1992;27:22–7.
7. Warden JW. *Grief counseling and grief therapy. a handbook for the mental health practitioner*. 4th ed. New York: Springer; 2009.
8. Franzini FR. Humor in therapy: the case for training therapists in its uses and risks. *J Gen Psychol* 2001;128:170–93.

9. Dolan RJ. Emotion, cognition, and behavior. *Science* 2002;298:1191–4.
10. Kinrade T, Hackson AC, Tomnay JE. The psychosocial needs of families during critical illness: comparison of nurses' and family members' perspectives. *Aust J Adv Nurs* 2009;27(1):82–8.
11. College of Intensive Care Medicine of Australia and New Zealand. *Guide to CICM training: trainees.* Melbourne, VIC: CICM; 2014. https://cicm.org.au.

8

Informed consent
Just sign here

The term informed consent first appeared in court documents in 1957, in a civil court ruling on the case of a patient named Martin Salgo. He went under anesthesia for what he thought was a routine procedure and woke up permanently paralyzed from the waist down. The doctor hadn't told him the procedure carried any risks at all.

Rebecca L. Skloot (1972–), US science and medicine writer, author of *The immortal life of Henrietta Lacks* (2010)[1]

*

Informed consent is a formal agreement given by a patient to undergo a proposed treatment. It also applies to the dying patient when considering relevant end-of-life treatment options. In an incapacitated patient, an advance care directive (ACD) or a substitute decision maker may give consent.

*

'We have a problem', Paul Constable said, sitting down by my desk in my office. 'Mrs King in bed 13. She's four days post tracheostomy. We removed her trachy tube five hours ago. She now has stridor and is coughing a fair bit – voice sounds hoarse.'

Mrs Anne King had arrived in the emergency department four days previously in severe breathing distress. She had acute epiglottitis or inflammation of the epiglottis – the cartilaginous flap at the base of the tongue that prevents aspiration of fluids and food into the trachea. Historically common in children two to four years old, the incidence is now rare (less than 1 : 100,000) in countries with mandatory vaccination against *Haemophilus influenzae* bacteria. The incidence in adults inexplicably remains constant, about twice that of children's, but nonetheless is still rare. Anne King presented with characteristic fever, swallowing difficulties, voice changes, drooling and breathing difficulties. It was a medical emergency; death would be swift if her airway became completely occluded.

With her airway at risk, an emergency operating theatre was immediately arranged. Anaesthetist Dr Larry O'Brien proceeded to secure her airway using a fibreoptic scope. This is a long, thin, flexible instrument with an eyepiece at the operator's end to view images through a lens at the distal tip. Dr O'Brien first loaded the fibrescope by passing its shaft through the lumen of a small endotracheal tube. With Anne King mildly sedated, he then inserted the fibrescope through her left nostril and visually navigated its tip past her nasal passages, mouth and swollen epiglottis, and between the vocal cords into her trachea. Finally, he 'railroaded' the endotracheal tube down the shaft of the fibrescope into the trachea. The endotracheal tube secured Anne King's airway, but its small diameter made spontaneous breathing arduous. Dr O'Brien then started general anaesthesia and Dr Hector Agonis, an ENT surgeon, performed a tracheostomy to insert a tracheostomy tube at her neck. It was a life-threatening scenario that was skillfully managed by the professional team.

'Stridor's not surprising, given her emergency airway manipulations', Paul continued. 'Probably temporary from swollen tissues, but laryngeal injury or vocal cord paralysis are considerations. She's distressed of course and angry.' He frowned and shook his head in sympathy. 'But not as angry as her husband, who vented his feelings at O'Brien, the anaesthetist, who came to see her. They kept saying that they were not told of this complication when giving informed consent for the tracheostomy. Shades of

Whitaker', he ended with a twist of drollness in his raised eyebrows.

*

What is informed consent?

Informed consent is a formal agreement given by a patient to undergo a proposed treatment (unless there is an 'exceptional' circumstance, see below). A doctor or health professional has a duty to disclose information to the patient who can then decide whether to receive or refuse the treatment. To be valid, the consent must be voluntary, informed, current and relevant to the treatment, and signed by the patient who is mentally competent. Informed consent, of course, also applies to treatment choices in end-of-life care, and is thus relevant in end-of-life considerations.

An informed consent is an acceptance of treatment based on a clear understanding of given information that is appropriate and adequate. In contrast, consent is simply an acceptance of treatment without necessarily being adequately informed of the implications and consequences of the treatment.

In informed consent, the patient is informed about the nature of the condition, the proposed treatment and who will deliver it, other options of care, the likely outcome of treatment, risks involved with the treatment and costs. There are many risks, major and minor, associated with most treatment, and it is not possible for any doctor to disclose every single one. What then should be disclosed? These are risks with severe outcomes (even if rare), common known risks (even if the adverse outcome is minor) and 'material' risks. These risks are 'material' if *the patient, as a reasonable person, would be likely to attach significance to the risk*, or *the doctor should reasonably be aware that the patient would be likely to attach significance to it*. The doctor should also provide any other information that the patient may ask, and be satisfied that the patient has understood the discussion.

Any medical procedure or treatment requires informed consent, be it surgical, medical, obstetric, imaging, investigational or a course of chemotherapy. Also, anaesthesia – whether general, regional, spinal or intravenous sedation – requires informed consent, as do all *invasive* treatments, including administration of blood or blood products and participation in ethics-approved research. In many jurisdictions, blood collection for measuring blood alcohol concentrations or diagnosing HIVs needs informed consent.

Legal basis for informed consent

Until the 1990s, Australian law followed the English approach of using the *Bolam principle* to determine medical negligence, based on the case of *Bolam v Friern Hospital Management* [1957].[2] Mr Bolam received electroconvulsive therapy with no muscle relaxant, during which he flailed and suffered injuries. He sued the hospital for negligence in not issuing relaxants, not restraining him and not disclosing the risks involved. Applying electroconvulsive therapy without muscle relaxants was the standard medical practice at the time, and the court ruled in favour of the hospital. The Bolam principle is that a health professional is not negligent if he or she acts according to a practice accepted at the time as proper by a responsible body of medical opinion, even though some other practitioners may adopt a different practice. Doctors would also rely on peer professional practice to determine the amount of information to disclose to their patients, even in getting consent to treatment.

The Bolam principle in defining the standard for informed consent and disclosure changed in Australia in 1992 following the High Court's decision on *Rogers v Whitaker*.[3] Maree Whitaker, who had been almost blind in her right eye, underwent elective surgery on that eye. The ophthalmologist, Dr Christopher Rogers, had advised her that surgery would improve the eye's appearance and would probably restore significant sight. He operated with skill and care but the procedure was unsuccessful, and she contracted a rare condition called *sympathetic ophthalmia* in her *left* eye, effectively leaving her completely blind. She sued Dr Rogers for negligence in the NSW Supreme Court, which eventually ended up in the High Court. He had not warned her of the risk of being rendered blind in both eyes. Although she had not specifically asked about the risk of *sympathetic ophthalmia* itself, she had expressed concern that her good left eye be not harmed. Dr Rogers argued that the Bolam principle should be applied to settle the issue. His peers would not normally have disclosed the risk of *sympathetic ophthalmia*, a rare complication occurring in only 1:14,000 procedures. The High Court found that Dr Rogers failed in his duty to disclose material risks inherent in the procedure. If Dr Rogers had informed Maree Whitaker of that risk, she would not have consented to the procedure, and the risk would not have materialised for her. The High Court's opinion on what should be disclosed has been reproduced by medical bodies such as the National Health and Medical Research Council (NHMRC) as general guidelines to help health professionals (*see Box 1*).[4]

---

1. Doctors Should Normally Discuss the Following Information

- The possible or likely nature of the illness or disease
- The proposed approach to investigation, diagnosis and treatment:
  - what the proposed approach entails
  - the expected benefits
  - common side effects and material risks of any intervention
  - whether the intervention is conventional or experimental
  - who will undertake the intervention
- Other options for investigation, diagnosis and treatment
- The degree of uncertainty of any diagnosis arrived at
- The degree of uncertainty about the therapeutic outcome
- The likely consequences of not choosing the proposed diagnostic procedure or treatment, or of not having any procedure or treatment at all
- Any significant long-term physical, emotional, mental, social, sexual or other outcome which may be associated with a proposed intervention
- The time involved
- The costs involved, including out-of-pocket costs

(Reproduced with permission from Australian National Health and Medical Research Council. *General guidelines for medical practitioners on providing information to patients*. Canberra: NHMRC; 1993)

Since *Rogers v Whitaker,* a number of courts in Australia have applied the standard of the case. Failure to disclose a material risk is not negligent by itself. Patients have to establish *causation:* the doctor failed in his duty of care to advise of a material risk; that failure to do so caused damage to the patient; and the patient, if informed of the risk beforehand, would not have consented to the procedure. Examples are: in *Dunning v Scheibner*[5] the plaintiff had tattoos removed from her back and arms by laser treatment and suffered severe pain and scarring, in *Tekanawa v Millican*[6] the plaintiff suffered unsightly scarring and abdominal pain after abdominoplasty or 'tummy-tuck' surgery, and in *Shaw v Langley*[7] there was scarring on Mrs Shaw's breasts and asymmetrical nipples following breast augmentation. Providing pamphlets and brochures about proposed procedures does not discharge the duty to adequately inform. The duty of care in providing advice on material risks is no less important when the proposed procedure is elective or non-therapeutic.

Rarity of a complication is no defence against lack of disclosure, as shown by *Rogers v Whitaker* and *Tai v Saxon*,[8] where the doctor failed to disclose the risk of a rectovaginal fistula following a hysterectomy, which had an incidence of $1:500$ procedures. Interestingly, in *Causer v Stafford-Bell*,[9] another case of rectovaginal fistula following hysterectomy ended in a different result because the plaintiff could not prove causation. In *Berger v Mutton*,[10] the plaintiff, a nurse, also could not prove causation. Her bowel was perforated when undergoing a gynaecological procedure. She alleged that she was not warned of the risk, and claimed that she would not have accepted that risk to consent to the procedure. The court found that her doctor had given warning of the associated risks, but she was determined to proceed to rule out the possibility of cancer. The court also doubted whether she could claim ignorance of the risks as she had substantial nursing and previous personal experience of a similar procedure.

Withdrawing treatment or withholding treatment does not require informed consent in Australia if the treatment is considered futile and burdensome and not in the patient's best interests (Chapter 6 Withdrawing treatment).

Informed consent in other jurisdictions

Disclosure of material risks is also the standard in some developed countries. In New Zealand, the Code of Health and Disability Services Consumers' Rights 1996 (Code of Rights)[11] contains this duty to inform of material risks. The UK adhered to the legal standard of its Bolam principle until 2015, following the Montgomery case.[12] Nadine Montgomery, a petite diabetic and mother of a child born with cerebral palsy, sued Lanarkshire Health Board. She argued that her obstetrician should have warned her of the particular risk to her and her baby of shoulder dystocia (a mechanical problem of obstructed shoulder) occurring during vaginal delivery. She had raised her concerns about vaginal delivery because of her petiteness, and argued that she should have been informed of the option of delivery by caesarean section, which would have avoided that risk and prevented her child's injury. The Supreme Court deemed the Bolam test to be unsuitable for discussing risks in her situation, as vaginal delivery in one so petite was not the accepted practice of a majority of peer obstetricians, and ruled in favour of the plaintiff on the basis of materiality of risks; the obstetrician should have given the fullest information or all possible options.

In the US, two legal standards can be applied, varying from state to state.[13] The 'reasonable practitioner' standard requires the doctor to disclose risks that would be disclosed by a reasonable practitioner in the relevant specialty. The second, the 'reasonable patient' standard, requires disclosure of risks that a reasonable patient would need to know to make an informed decision. To adhere to those standards, the risks to be disclosed could be 'material' to the patient's decision making.

*

I met with Jason King alone in the interview room. He was an overweight man, fortyish in age and of medium height. He was a property developer and his tan suit, pink shirt with a white collar and red polka dot tie exuded loud wealth.

'I'm sorry for what Anne and you went through', I started off. 'ENT has just seen her and her vocal cords and epiglottis are back to normal now. She had paresis or partial paralysis of her left vocal cord. We don't know what caused it, but bruising of the tissues in the larynx and / or nearby nerves from the emergency airway procedures is the likely cause. Anyway, she's well now and we will send her to the ENT ward shortly, and she should be able to go home the next day or two.'

He listened attentively. 'Good. Thank you. She's a keen singer you know. Member of "Sweet Adelines", the Barbershop singers? She would have been devastated if her voice had changed.' He looked sideways, thoughtful. 'We were angry, very angry … not at you guys', he hastily added, raising a conciliatory right hand. 'Just the anaesthetist and surgeon. They did not tell us about the risk of vocal cord damage.'

'I understand', I said. 'Normally anaesthesia and ENT would complete their consent process, using their own specialty's *procedure specific consent form* that would have covered the risks of laryngeal and vocal cord damage, but the anaesthetist and surgeon were busy in theatre. The emergency department doctor completed consent using the general template form designed for emergencies. You realise that your wife almost died? It was a real emergency. In my opinion, the anaesthetist saved Anne's life.'

He raised his forehead in surprise, his jaws gaping. He did not know what I had told him. I knew that he was not present when she arrived by ambulance.

'My company's lawyers briefed me on failure to inform risks', he persisted. '*Rogers v Whitaker*? The closest case to Anne's, I was told, was *Chappel v Hart* where the lady lost her voice. You know that one.' He had sought legal advice as we had anticipated.

'The Chappel case was different. It was chest surgery and elective. Anne's was an emergency tracheostomy', I said, thinking *his company's lawyers are specialists in conveyancing, not litigation.* 'Obtaining consent in medical emergencies is different from that in elective procedures.'

*

In an emergency where a person is incapable of giving consent, treatment that is necessary to save a person's life or prevent serious injury may be provided without consent if the patient does not have an ACD or substitute decision maker readily available (Chapter 3 Advance care directives). However, if the person is able to provide consent, the doctors should still seek consent (albeit somewhat abridged due to time pressures).

Elective treatment proposed for patients who lack capacity, requires consent via an ACD or substitute decision maker. ACDs generally override decisions by substitute decision makers. Most jurisdictions recognise a hierarchy of decision makers (*see Box 2*).

2. Hierarchy of Decision Makers
• Advance care directive
• Enduring guardian – chosen by the individual
• Guardian – appointed by the state
• Spouse or de facto partner
• Adult son or daughter
• Parent
• Sibling
• Primary unpaid caregiver
• Other person with a close personal relationship

For a child (under the age of 18 years), apart from life-threatening emergencies, a doctor must obtain the consent of a parent before undertaking treatment. Depending on circumstances, consent may also be given by a guardian, the court and, in many jurisdictions, the child. If the doctor establishes that a child has sufficient maturity to make decisions regarding their own treatment, the consent of the child alone is sufficient consent to that treatment. This is known as a 'mature minor' or 'Gillick competence',[14] and there is no defined age at which a child can consent to medical treatment. Patients with mental illness are also considered differently. Specific laws of jurisdictions govern treatment of such patients.

Jason King likened his wife's circumstances to *Chappel v Hart*,[15] but that case was entirely different. Mrs Hart underwent an elective upper chest operation to remove a pouch in her oesophagus that caused problems with swallowing. Dr Chappel performed the operation without negligence but perforated the oesophagus, which led to mediastinitis. This infection of mid-chest tissues damaged the laryngeal nerve, causing the paralysis of her right vocal cord that altered her voice. Dr Chappel had warned her of the risk of perforation but not of the complication of vocal cord damage. The High Court – by a 3 : 2 majority – upheld the decision of the NSW Supreme Court that he was liable, in that he breached his duty in failure to warn of this risk. Mrs Hart did not contend that, had Dr Chappel warned her of this risk, she would have decided against surgery. Instead, she claimed that, had she known, she would have had the operation at another time, probably with a more experienced surgeon. The Court found that if she had been properly warned she would have taken a different course of action (i.e. surgery at a later date by another surgeon), which may have averted the injury. However, this decision of 'failure to warn' as a *prima facie* case of causation raises an evidentiary difficulty. There was no evidence that another surgeon performing the same surgery at a later date would never perforate the oesophagus. Mrs Hart had not strictly proved causation, at odds with the onus in previous cases of negligence after *Rogers v Whitaker*.

*

There was a knock on my door. Rosemary Smith opened the door and stuck her head in. 'You know the *Palladium*, the new hotel-entertainment complex? It's having its grand opening next week – fireworks, concert, food, drinks. The wannabes would give their right arm to be invited. The owner's Jason King, husband of Anne King. Remember them? Guess what? He's just sent us 50 free invitations to the event. I hear that Dr Agonis and Dr O'Brien got invitations too.'

⁎

Reflections

- Doctors must obtain informed consent in all relevant procedures.
- Doctors must be cognisant of what constitute material risks.
- Patients and substitute decision makers should think of all possible material risks associated with the proposed procedure, and raise them when considering whether to accept the treatment.
- Doctors, patients and substitute decision makers should consider other options of treatment and their consequences.
- Doctors must inform the patient or the substitute decision maker of the implications and consequences if they refuse any proposed treatment.
- Patients and substitute decision makers should ask questions on anything that they are unsure about.
- Informed consent forms must be recorded, as should all discussions pertinent to the proposed procedure.
- Patients should prepare an advance care directive and nominate their substitute decision maker before undergoing a major procedure.

References

1. Skloot RL. *The immortal life of Henrietta Lacks.* New York: Crown; 2010.
2. *Bolam v Friern Barnet Hospital Management Committee* [1957] 1 WLR 582.
3. *Rogers v Whitaker* [1992] 175 CLR 479.
4. Australian National Health and Medical Research Council. *General guidelines for medical practitioners on providing information to patients.* Canberra: NHMRC; 1993. p. 11.
5. Unreported, NSW Sup Ct 15 February 1994.
6. Unreported, Qld Dist Ct 11 February 1994.
7. Unreported, Qld Dist Ct 24 November 1993.

8. WASC 1 March 1996.

9. ACTSC 90, 14 November 1997.

10. Unreported, NSW Dist Ct 22 November 1994.

11. Health and Disability Commissioner. *Code of Health and Disability Services Consumers' Rights 1996 (Code of Rights)*. HDC, New Zealand. https://www.hdc.org.nz/your-rights/about-the-code/code-of-health-and-disability-services-consumers-rights/.

12. *Montgomery v Lanarkshire Health Board* [2015] SC 11 [2015] 1 AC 1430.

13. Johnson LJ. Malpractice: your informed consent may not be good enough. *Medscape* 2011; Feb 10. https://www.medscape.com/viewarticle/736411_2.

14. Skene L. Consent to medical procedures in children. In: Skene L, editor. *Law and medical practice – rights, duties, claims and defences*. 3rd ed. Chatswood, NSW, Australia: LexisNexis Butterworth; 2008.

15. HCA 55 2 September 1998 – 195 CLR 232; 72 ALJR 1344; 156 ALR 157.

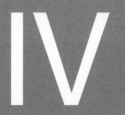

Death

Brain death and vegetative states

Dead or alive

Right now, the economy is a whole lot like a fairly good-looking brain-dead chick in a persistent vegetative coma. You can't really wake her up, but there's things she's still good for.[1]

Cintra Wilson (1967–), American writer, satirist and cultural critic

Either he's dead or my watch has stopped.

Groucho Marx (1890–1977), American comedian, writer, actor,
TV star in *A Day at the Races*, a 1937 film

*

Historically, death was defined as irreversible cessation of breathing and heartbeat (Chapter 2 Ethics in death and dying). Today, brain death is the other definition of death. Brain death is the irreversible, complete loss of brain function activity necessary to sustain life, the consequence of a devastating neurological injury in different forms. These include traumatic brain injury, a stroke caused by a ruptured or occluded blood vessel in the brain, and anoxia if the heart has stopped and the brain is deprived of oxygen.

*

'You know, of course, that the patient must be in coma for at least four hours, with evidence of intracranial pathology. You start by excluding factors that can affect cranial nerve reflexes, the *preconditions*. You cannot proceed to test for brain death if the patient records *any* abnormal reading in body temperature, blood pressure, blood sugar level and serum electrolytes … or has a metabolic or endocrine disorder. Neuromuscular function must be intact', I told Dr Rachel Lim. We were at the bedside of Andy Giff, with his nurse Sheila looking on. I was about to conduct a second set of clinical brain death tests to diagnose brain death, and thus declare death.[2] Milton Franks had completed the first set three hours ago.

For a 17-year-old, Andy looked small lying in bed, his head swathed in bandages almost hiding his brain-monitoring leads. Other leads and tubing on his tanned chest and arms connected him to monitors above his head and to fluid infusion pumps. A tracheal tube delivered breaths from the ventilator. Around the tube, his lips and chin had a faint fuzz of adolescent facial hair. A dozen get-well cards and a teddy bear decked in a purple jumper emblazoned with 'DOCKERS' – the club of his Aussie Rules football heroes – sat on the shelf above the electrical, gas and suction outlets.

*

Brain death

The brain comprises the *cerebrum*, the *cerebellum* and the *brainstem*. The cerebrum or cortex is the largest part, associated with higher brain function such as thought and action. At the back and bottom of the cerebrum, the cerebellum is important in cognition, coordination, equilibrium and posture. At the bottom, the brainstem connects the cerebrum and the spinal cord, and relays signals between them through neurons called cranial nerve nuclei. The brainstem controls basic body functions such as breathing, swallowing, heart rate, blood pressure, consciousness and wakefulness.

Some jurisdictions define brain death as death of the brainstem, and others as death of the whole brain including the brainstem. There is no obvious difference between whole-brain death and brainstem death to denote death. In both there is unconsciousness, absence of any response to stimulation, absence of spontaneous breathing and no chance of recovery. The difference lies in the results of testing. Bedside clinical tests are necessary and sufficient to diagnose brainstem death. Some doctors may include an EEG (electroencephalogram) or a blood-flow study after clinical brainstem death has been confirmed. If they show total absence of EEG activity or blood flow, whole-brain death is then diagnosed. These extra tests are confirmatory and not diagnostic. They may otherwise show residual electrical and / or flow activity in *some* cells, which are not indicative of brain function. Even a heart that stops beating has cells with residual electrical activity. The diagnosis of brainstem death remains unchanged, and there is no chance of recovering consciousness or breathing.

Technically, if the cerebrum (the 'thinking brain') is dead and the brainstem is not, life can be sustained, but without any cognitive abilities, as exemplified in the bizarre story of Mike the headless chicken (*see Box*).

Mike the Headless Chicken

In its 22 October 1945 issue, US *Life* magazine reported that a poor Colorado farmer had beheaded a chicken but it refused to die, and it continued to walk unsteadily. Most of its skull had been chopped off, but its brainstem and an ear were left. Mike the headless chicken lived for 18 months, being fed with an eye-dropper, earning income for its owner as a sideshow attraction. It finally succumbed by choking.

BRAIN DEATH CONCEPT

With increasing developments in resuscitation, life support and organ donation, the medical and legal professions in the late 1960s and 1970s looked for definitions of death more specific than cessation of heartbeat and breathing. Harvard Medical School published a report in 1968 to define irreversible coma that led towards consensus considerations of brain death. The Conference of Medical Colleges in UK published, in 1976[3] and 1979,[4] diagnostic criteria of brainstem death, and in 1995 the UK Royal College of Physicians defined death based on the irreversible loss of brainstem function alone.[5] In 1981 the US approved the *Uniform Determination of Death* Act,[6] which defined death as death of the whole brain including the brainstem, and which has since been recognised by all states. Brain death today is accepted as legal death in many countries including Australia. In 1977 the Australian Law Reform Commission published two definitions of brain death: *irreversible cessation of circulation of blood in the body of a person – circulatory death*, or *irreversible cessation of all function of the brain of a person – brain death*. Brain death is determined according to accepted medical standards. In Australia, this is by clinical criteria as described for Andy Giff, or by special imaging techniques.

*

I was on duty four days earlier when we admitted Andy into the ICU. He was riding a bicycle on a suburban road when he swerved into the path of a car to avoid a wayfaring cat. The driver could not miss him and Andy sustained head injuries, fractured ribs and a broken left leg. He did not wear a helmet. Resuscitated in the emergency department, he arrived in ICU with a secure airway and a set of computed tomography (CT) films. The films showed skull fractures, brain contusions and haemorrhages and generalised diffuse swelling, consistent with the impact of his head hitting the road. He remained unconscious.

A consultant neurosurgeon, Dr Gordon Wong, had seen Andy. Gordon was a small quiet man, always smartly dressed and unusually modest for a surgeon. In his calm way, he completed a neurological examination on Andy, and walked briskly to the imaging viewing boxes to look at the films. He scrutinised each one, occasionally peering closely, and finally turned to me, grimaced and shook his head. 'Not good', he said, his way of expressing concern.

We met later with Andy's parents. Gordon spoke to them and stressed his concern – the expected development of cerebral oedema or brain swelling. 'The skull's a rigid box', he said. 'Like any injured tissue, the brain will swell, a normal body response. The swelling compresses brain tissue and blood vessels. Blood flow then decreases and reduces oxygen supply to the brain.' He explained that he would insert a device in Andy's skull to monitor his intracranial pressure. It was a lot of information for the distraught couple to absorb. Gordon had anticipated their agonising question. 'I use the term "guarded prognosis" at this stage', he said. 'Andy has a severe head injury and may die from brain swelling. But he's young and we have had good results with traumatic brain injury in young people.' He did not mention the sequelae of neurological impairment that would follow if Andy were to survive.

*

Sheila, Andy's nurse, was a small, attractive nurse on a working holiday from Ireland. 'Andy's BP', she said in her glorious Irish lilt, 'has been drifting down in the past hour.' She nodded towards the monitor above Andy's head. The digital blood pressure reading showed a low '80:50'.

I made a brief physical examination and said, 'I'll start the brain death testing now.' I used my pen to exert a force on Andy's shins. 'Coma is unresponsive. Let's test his cranial nerves', I said to Rachel Lim who was writing down my findings. I proceeded to test the integrity of the cranial nerve reflexes that pass through the brainstem. The cranial nerves did not respond to stimuli, indicating brainstem death. Finally, I disconnected him from the ventilator to test apnoea or absence of spontaneous breathing. As a safety measure, we had changed his oxygen supply to 100% before our tests. Andy did not breathe and, after 10 minutes, I reconnected him to the ventilator.

'This is the second test, and that confirms brain death. Time of death...', I said, looking at my watch, '... is 10.43 a.m. I'll speak to his family.' We stood together, silent in our thoughts, looking down at Andy, dead at 17.

*

BRAIN DEATH TESTING

In Australia, brain death cannot be verified unless there is evidence of severe brain injury sufficient to cause death and other causes of deep coma have been excluded, such as drugs and abnormal blood sugar and blood electrolyte levels. These are the *preconditions*. There must also be a minimum of four hours observation on mechanical ventilation, during which the patient is completely unresponsive to all stimuli. Various brainstem cranial nerves have reflex reactions (or responses) to sensory stimulation such as pain, cold and heat. In clinical testing, the responses below are *all* absent in brainstem death.

- *Pupillary reflex:* pupils do not respond to light, and remain fixed and dilated.
- *Cold caloric eye reflex:* injecting ice-cold water into an ear canal elicits no eye movement. This normally triggers rapid eye movements called nystagmus.
- *Corneal reflex:* touching the cornea with cotton wool elicits no eye blink.
- *Gag reflex:* touching the back of the throat with a spatula elicits no gagging.
- *Cough reflex:* stimulating the trachea with a suction catheter elicits no coughing.
- *Apnoea test:* absence of spontaneous breathing when disconnected from the ventilator.

Clinical testing also mandates separate testing by two different specialists. Some doctors use confirmatory EEG or blood-flow studies after clinical brainstem death has been confirmed. Apart from qualifying brain death as whole-brain death rather than as brainstem death, these extra tests are not essential.

*

Bill and Mona Giff and their two adult offspring were waiting in the interview room. The parents were well dressed, in their late forties. Mona sat between their eldest, Jacob and Andy's older sister Jenny, both in their twenties. Bill sat next to his son, and the men stood up when I entered the room. I shook hands with them and moved my chair closer to them. They sat stiffly, faces lined with worry, expecting the worse. Sheila walked in and sat a discreet distance away; another nurse was substituting for her at the bedside.

'Thank you for coming in. Remember what we spoke about yesterday? What do you know about Andy's condition now?', I asked. I did not want to speak on different planes if they had misunderstood aspects of Andy's care.

Mona and her offspring looked at each other, and then to Bill. 'We understood that Andy's got low blood pressure', Bill said.

'Yes, we had started Andy on inotropic drugs … heart stimulants.' I glanced at Sheila. She nodded and gave the family a restrained smile, hoping to reassure them and perhaps project some comfort. Mona let out a big breath.

'I had previously told you yesterday that Andy's brain was swollen and his intracranial pressure was high. His lungs, oxygenation and other organ systems were good, though. But his condition deteriorated last night. I'm sorry but I'm afraid I have bad news now', I said.

The Giffs looked stunned. Before I could continue, Bill spoke. 'You did mention yesterday brain death and … testing Andy?'

'Yes. His condition deteriorated overnight', I repeated. 'We then conducted the brain death tests I mentioned yesterday. Twice, over three hours ago and just now.' I chose my words, 'Andy's prognosis, as Dr Wong and I had mentioned to you, was always poor. I'm sorry but Andy will not recover now', I said and paused before continuing. 'Both sets of tests showed Andy to be brain dead. Andy is now legally dead.' A sense of gloom descended on the room. Mona gave a sudden sob. Jacob and Jenny leaned towards her to hold her hands.

'He should have worn his helmet!', Mona exclaimed, her fists clutching tissues, a mother in anguish. We kept silent. I handed her more tissues, and she sobbed as she wiped her eyes.

Jenny sniffed and reached forward to pluck a handful of tissues. She remained silent, then said suddenly, 'I don't want Andy to die.' She took a deep breath and continued. 'Surely something … anything … you doctors can do something? He's not dead. He's still breathing. He looks pink … alive. Just continue the ventilator. He'll pull through.'

Jacob, who had been comforting his mother, lifted his head to look at me. 'He was on his way to see his mate just down our street. Ours is a quiet street. No need to wear a helmet there just to go….' Mona started to cry again. Jacob stopped and turned back to his mother.

'Would a helmet have lessened Andy's head injury?', Bill asked. This issue was troubling them, but he did not say 'Would it have saved his life?'

'Would you wear one?', Jacob abruptly asked.

'Yes. And I always do.' I did not elaborate, not wanting to add to their grief. I changed tack. 'We carried out two brain death tests. They are true and valid. Properly conducted, among thousands, no test in the world over the past 30 years has been shown to be false. Brain death is legally also death. I am so sorry but Adam is legally dead. Even if we continue with ventilation and life support treatment, his heart will eventually stop spontaneously, in hours or one to two days. As is the practice, we will soon stop all treatment. Are there any family members you wish to contact before we do so?', I asked. Bill shook his head. The family had moved from Durban, South Africa. They had no other relatives in Australia.

*

IS THE BRAIN-DEAD PATIENT ON LIFE SUPPORT STILL ALIVE?

The answer to this perennial question is 'no'. The brain-dead patient cannot breathe by himself. Mechanical ventilation provides oxygen to his heart, which continues to beat, and the patient looks 'pink and asleep'. Despite continuing ventilatory support, the heartbeat will eventually stop because of complete 'system failure'. The dead brainstem can no longer control cardiac activity. This may take hours or a few days. The condition of brain death is different to that of persistent vegetative state (see below). The first quotation to introduce this chapter is as crass as it is wrong in fact. No patient with brain death has ever recovered spontaneous breathing or mental or voluntary body function.

*

'There is one more matter I must raise. I'm sorry but it's also my job to raise organ donation with you', I said to the Giff family when there was an urgent-sounding knock on the door. Andy's locum bed nurse stuck her head through the door and gestured to me to follow her. Sheila and I immediately left the Giff family to go to Andy's bed. Andy's blood pressure had fallen drastically. The inotropic infusion was not having any effect. His heart was giving up. We quickly ushered his family to the bedside. I did not, could not, broach the subject of organ donation again at this moment. Andy suffered a cardiac arrest 30 minutes later. We did not stop treatment but we did not attempt CPR. The ECG had flat-lined and alarms sounded. I could feel no pulse. We had been spared the duty to stop his mechanical ventilation before his cardiac death. Sheila drew the bed curtains, and we left the family with Adam. Later, Sheila laid out Adam in death, helped by her nursing colleagues. Then, in the staff room, she burst out crying, and later sought comfort from the hospital's Catholic chaplain.

I saw the Giffs after they had said their goodbyes. They were waiting in the corridor. Bill shook my hand and Mona gave me a hug. Jacob comforted Jenny, her head on his shoulder. They were quiet with red puffy eyes, exhausted in grief. I said nothing. The death of a young patient – '*a bright future snuffed out*' – always hits everyone hard. I find it hard to ascribe goodness and dignity to some deaths, only sadness always.

*

Traumatic injury is the leading cause of death of Australians under 45 years, accounting for 25% of hospital admissions. About 1000 victims sustain traumatic brain injury each year, at enormous financial costs to the nation. *Why didn't Andy wear a helmet?* It's mandatory in Australia. Data tends to support wearing of helmets to reduce the risk of head injury. Different safety records among countries may be explained by disparate factors such as education, traffic density, cycling infrastructure (e.g. dedicated bicycle lanes), communal attitude to cyclists, and the culture of motorised road users (e.g. drink driving and road rage behaviours). Denmark and the Netherlands have a low helmet use with among the best bicycle safety records, but their culture of road users is very different to that of Australia's. Indeed, studies report that unhelmeted cyclists are at greater risk in the road environment of Australia.[7,8] Also, some cyclist injuries and deaths are caused by falling onto the road or kerb, and not by collision with motor vehicles. Helmets, then, offer better protection against severe head injury.

Anti-helmet groups say that mandatory helmet use discourages cycling, encourages riskier riding behaviour, shifts responsibility to the cyclist and removes an individual's right of choice. These are ludicrous arguments. Surely one has to accept that riding a bicycle carries a risk of head injury, albeit small. Then, like cricket, motor racing, skiing, skateboarding or any activity that has a potential – no matter how small – for head injury, wearing a helmet is surely a no-brainer. This, to avert potential death or permanent brain disability, is a small nuisance we can easily endure. Like chronic smoking, 'it's my right to do so' is also 'it's your wasted death for what?' The taxpayer of course, picks up the big tab for the ensuing hospital care that could have been avoided.

BRAIN DEATH AND COMA

The media and the public often confuse brain death with coma and vegetative states. They use the wrong terms interchangeably to describe disordered consciousness, but these conditions have different prognoses and outcomes. Differentiation of these diagnoses is important for principles of bedside care and healthcare policy.[9,10] Coma is a profound state of 'eyes-closed' unconsciousness. The patient is alive and *able to breathe spontaneously*, but does not move or respond to the stimuli. Coma is the initial presentation of severe brain injury from any cause and is self-limited, lasting for hours or days. A comatose state can progress to different possible outcomes depending on the cause: brain death, vegetative state, minimally conscious state, intellectual impairment or complete recovery. The prognosis of each depends on the cause, patient age and current duration. Hypoxic or oxygen-deprived injury has the worst prognosis.

Persistent vegetative state

The term *persistent vegetative state* or PVS describes 'wakeful unresponsiveness' in patients with *open* eyes but no awareness of self, others or the environment. They cannot think or reason (with no cognitive or higher-brain function), but they retain autonomic functions such as spontaneous breathing and circulation, unlike in brain death. They may move spontaneously, open their eyes to stimuli and cry, laugh or grimace occasionally, but they do not speak, understand or respond to commands. There is no control over bladder or bowels. The vegetative state is labelled persistent if it lasts over a month, and permanent after 3–12 months. PVS is often confused with coma and with brain death.

To add to further confusion over disordered consciousness, a new clinical entity is now recognised: *minimally conscious state* or MCS. This is a state of consciousness with fluctuating minimal awareness of self and surroundings. Such patients may gesture, say words or phrases and even display patterns of intention and memory, but these actions may be fleeting and inconsistent. Prognosis can be open ended. MCS may progress to PVS;

improvement ('emergence') is possible but rare. In the US, two cases were reported to have recovered fluent speech after 9 and 19 years respectively of confirmed MCS.

The diagnoses of PVS and MCS are made by structured assessments by experts. There are no diagnostic biochemical or imaging tests. Application of the term 'permanent' implies that recovery is unlikely. Confirmation of the diagnosis is important to consider treatment plans. Decisions to withdraw tube feeding and hydration in a patient diagnosed as permanent vegetative state have ethical and legal implications. The prolonged legal battles in the United States to withdraw feeding and hydration from Nancy Cruzan and Terri Schiavo, and from Tony Bland in the UK, are well known (Chapter 6 Withdrawing treatment). Similar considerations also apply to withholding life-sustaining medications. Carers should obtain legal advice, and must respect advance care directives in the patient's best interests.

*

Reflections

- Lay people, especially journalists, and doctors (yes even some doctors) should understand the difference between brain death, coma and vegetative states.
- Brain death is legal death. Doctors need not seek consent to stop treatment.
- There is no recovery of any form or function from brain death.
- Continuing 'life support' (mechanical ventilation) is futile in brain death. The heart will eventually stop beating, despite continuing full life support treatment.

References

1. Wilson C. *Caligula for president: better American living through tyranny*. New York: Bloomsbury; 2010.
2. Australian and New Zealand Intensive Care Society. *The ANZICS statement on death and organ donation*, ed. 3.2. Camberwell, VIC: ANZICS; 2013. https://anzics.com.au.
3. Diagnosis of brain death. Statement issued by the honorary secretary of the Conference of Medical Royal Colleges and their Faculties in the United Kingdom on 11 October 1976. *BMJ* 1976;2:1187–8.

4. Diagnosis of death. Memorandum issued by the honorary secretary of the Conference of Medical Royal Colleges and their Faculties in the United Kingdom on 15 January 1979. *BMJ* 1979;1:332.

5. [no authors listed]. Criteria for the diagnosis of brain stem death. Review of a working group convened by the Royal College of Physicians, endorsed by the Conference of Medical Royal Colleges and their Faculties in the United Kingdom. *J R Coll Physicians Lond* 1995;29(5):381–2.

6. *Uniform Determination of Death Act 1981*. Chicago, IL: Uniform Law Commission; 1981.

7. Beck B, Cameron PA, Fitzgerald MC, Judson RT, Teague W, Lyons RA, et al. Road safety: serious injuries remain a major unsolved problem. *Med J Aust* 2017;207(6):244–9.

8. Dinh M, Curtis K, Ivers R. The effectiveness of helmets in reducing head injuries and hospital treatment costs: a multicentre study. *Med J Aust* 2013;198:415–17.

9. Royal College of Physicians. *Prolonged disorders of consciousness: national clinical guidelines*. London: Royal College of Physicians; 2015. https://rcplondon.ac.uk.

10. Fins JJ. Brain injury: the vegetative and minimally conscious states. In: Crowley M, editor. *From birth to death and bench to clinic: the Hastings Center bioethics briefing book for journalists, policymakers, and campaigns*. Garrison, NY: The Hastings Center; 2008. pp. 15–20, [Chapter 4].

10

Euthanasia

Good death or bad death?

With daggers, bodkins, bullets, man can make
a bruise or break of exit for his life,
but is that a quietus, O tell me, is it quietus?

D.H. Lawrence (1885–1930), Playwright, poet, author,
in 'The ship of death' (1929)[1]

*

Euthanasia is one of the most debated issues in modern societies, and it presents ethical, moral, legal and medical dilemmas. The topic is relevant in discussions on end-of-life care, as some propose it to be a vehicle in life's last extraordinary journey.

*

'Euthanasia. It was euthanasia!', Dr Ryan Patel from the department of vascular surgery exclaimed, staring defiantly at the audience of his peers. It was a peer review meeting, held jointly every month by the department of intensive care, the department of anaesthesia and all the surgical departments. A medical audit meeting, each department took turns to present three selected cases, review decisions on treatment and make recommendations

123

to improve care. Dr Patel was presenting the case of Mrs CJ, 83 years old with known heart disease, who had arrived in the emergency department in profound shock from a leaking abdominal aortic aneurysm ('triple A', a ruptured aorta in the abdomen). Her blood pressure was barely recordable even after massive blood transfusions. He was keen to operate on her, but the duty anaesthetist had refused to anaesthetise, and intensive care had refused to admit into ICU. Dr Patel finally accused the two departments of the act of euthanasia, a criminal offence.

*

What is euthanasia?

Euthanasia is a powder-keg issue that, once lit, sets off an explosive debate between advocates and opponents. The word 'euthanasia' originates from the Greek word *euthanatos*, meaning 'easy death'. Euthanasia, in concept, represents the process of ending the life of an individual who has a terminal illness with unbearable pain and suffering. However, the term 'euthanasia' has had different meanings depending on usage, as reflected by past practices reviewed briefly below. Common to all past practices was the intention to deliberately terminate life.

History of euthanasia

The origins of euthanasia can be traced back to Ancient Greece and Rome. Plato (428 to 348 BCE), Socrates (470 to 399 BCE) and Seneca the Elder (54 BCE to CE 39) supported euthanasia and suicide; indeed Socrates' death was self-inflicted by swallowing the poison hemlock. The practice of euthanasia persisted despite opposition by Hippocrates (460 to 370 BCE); his Hippocratic Oath included not prescribing 'a lethal drug to cause death to please someone'. Ancient Greek and Roman cultures did not revere the sanctity of life, and infanticide, abortion, killing of the 'mentally feeble' and euthanasia were common practices. With the spread of Judaism and Christianity in the first millennium – with their beliefs in the sanctity of life and the worth of the individual – euthanasia became increasingly rejected. This was a massive change, and other world religions – Buddhism, Islam and Hinduism

– similarly viewed killing oneself or another to relieve misery was wrong. This view remained through the Middle Ages to the mid 17th century. The 'Age of Enlightenment', the 17th- and 18th-century intellectual movement in Europe, emphasised reason, individualism and scepticism. Enlightenment thinkers challenged traditional religious views, including laws on suicide and euthanasia. However, the masses once again turned to traditional Judeo-Christian views after the Enlightenment with the help of church leaders and Victorian evangelicalism.

In the modern age, euthanasia emerged and hit a pinnacle in Germany during the Nazi era. It started in 1920 with a book *The release of the destruction of life devoid of value*[2] by two Germans, Karl Binding (a lawyer) and Alfred Hoche (a doctor), who argued for euthanasia. They offered compassion as the reason, but they also advocated euthanasia for mentally retarded children they described as 'useless idiots'. Hitler enthusiastically adopted that view. From 1936 he enacted euthanasia programs to exterminate those with incurable illness, physical handicaps and mental disorders, including children. In World War II the Nazis extended the euthanasia programs to 'inferior races' – Jews, Gypsies, Russians and Poles – as well as homosexuals, the aged and political prisoners. His killing of millions was done not for compassion, but rather to socially engineer a perfect German Aryan race.

Definition of euthanasia

With different purposes of ending life by an intended intervention, what then is euthanasia? This book offers this definition: '*A deliberate and direct action, with known intent, to end the life of a terminally ill patient with unbearable pain and suffering and at the patient's request.*' This definition has four elements: a deliberate intervention, intentionality (to cause death), conditions of incurable illness and intractable suffering, and voluntary request. The motive is accepted to be good, the intervention to be painless and the outcome to be beneficial to the patient.

The debate on euthanasia is compounded when the elements of terminal illness, intractable suffering and even voluntary request are considered non-vital, as history relates. *Involuntary euthanasia* (against the will) is unacceptable; such deaths are murder[3] in any civilised jurisdiction. *Non-voluntary euthanasia*, when consent is not available, such as for comatose or demented patients or children – labelled 'mercy killing' – is similarly unacceptable, despite any good intention to end the subject's suffering. It breaches the ethical principles of autonomy and consent, and is homicide under common law in Australia and other countries. Hence considerations of legalising euthanasia must apply only to voluntary euthanasia – that is, that requested by the patient.

Terminology or classification

Different terms have been ascribed to practices of 'euthanasia' that add to confusion. 'Euthanasia' is often offered as an umbrella term with two broad groups: *active* euthanasia and *passive* euthanasia, each with '*voluntary*' and '*non-voluntary*' divisions (*see Box*). As explained above, any non-voluntary and involuntary forms of 'euthanasia' are unacceptable.

Classification/Terminology Used for Euthanasia

- Active voluntary euthanasia – doctor administered
- Active non-voluntary euthanasia – mercy killing[a]
- Active assisted suicide – self-administered euthanasia
- Passive voluntary euthanasia – death from refusing life-saving treatment[b]
- Passive non-voluntary euthanasia – withdrawing or withholding futile treatment[b] or withdrawing treatment in brain death[b]

[a]Unacceptable.
[b]Irrelevant.

Passive voluntary euthanasia is a term sometimes given to a death from refusing treatment. In developed countries, medical treatment requires informed consent from the patient (Chapter 8 Informed consent). The patient may, however, exercise his or her right of *autonomy* and refuse to consent to treatment, or request the withdrawal of treatment already started. This right is paramount, even if the treatment offered is life saving. Respect of such wishes is good medical practice and compliance currently occurs in Australia under various circumstances and scenarios. The patient dies shortly afterwards from the underlying disease process, and the death is not euthanasia. The patient requested an omission of treatment, with no deliberate, active action to cause death. Thus '*passive voluntary euthanasia*' is an irrelevant classification.

The term *passive non-voluntary euthanasia* has been given to a death following withdrawing or withholding futile treatment. Doctors do not have a duty to prolong life at all costs. If a treatment does not offer a reasonable hope of benefit, and if it imposes unacceptable burdens on the patient, that treatment is not warranted. Futile treatment can be withdrawn or withheld (Chapter 6 Withdrawing treatment), and this is universally practised, especially in end-of-life scenarios. Death inevitably follows; it is due to the underlying disease and not to any premeditated action to terminate life. Similarly, stopping treatment when brain death is diagnosed (Chapter 9 Brain death and vegetative states) is not passive euthanasia. Thus *passive non-voluntary euthanasia* is another irrelevant classification that can create confusion and fear. Dr Patel was incorrect in calling the decision on Mrs C 'euthanasia'.

From the above considerations, euthanasia is voluntary and an active act. It follows that euthanasia has two scenarios:

1. Active voluntary euthanasia – *doctor-administered*
   The patient wishes to die and requests the doctor for assistance, who then performs the act to kill, usually as an injection of lethal drugs. In jurisdictions in which euthanasia is illegal, the person who complies with that patient's request to knowingly end life commits homicide.
2. Active assisted suicide – *patient-administered* or 'assisted suicide'
   The patient wishes to die and requests the doctor for assistance, who then provides the means (such as advice, drugs and apparatus), but the patient performs the deadly act. Although suicide or attempted suicide is no longer a criminal act in Australia, assisting suicide is a crime in Australian states and many countries.

Doctrine of double effect

Discussions on euthanasia often raise the *doctrine of double effect*. It is an ethical principle in medicine that permits an act intended for a beneficial effect, but which may cause an otherwise undesirable, unintended effect. For example, pain associated with a terminal illness may require increasing doses of opioid medications. This will suppress the patient's breathing and may thus hasten death, but the primary goal is to relieve pain and suffering, and not to effect death – a subtle but huge difference. Four conditions must apply to justify the act:

1. The nature of the act is good.
2. The bad effect is not the means to achieve the good effect.
3. The intention is to achieve the good effect, with the bad effect being an unintended side effect.
4. The good effect is considered to outweigh the bad effect to justify causing the bad effect.

Although the acceptable amount of pain medications and the meaning of 'hastens death' are legal grey areas, the death is not considered euthanasia in palliative care practice and in specified laws in the UK, South Australia, Western Australia and Queensland.

Countries with legalised euthanasia

Victoria was the first and only Australian state to legalise patient-assisted euthanasia in 2017, to take effect in 2019. Euthanasia is legal in some countries. Jurisdictions where euthanasia is legal generally impose common strict criteria to comply, for example:

- an incurable medical condition (illness or disease which may include disability; some jurisdictions specify terminal illness)
- an enduring, intolerable suffering to the individual
- an expectation to live for a limited time period, say six months
- informed consent as a written declaration, and
- competency to make the decision.
  Common procedural safeguards include:
- two independent doctors – with some laws specifying a psychiatrist – must agree that a patient is eligible
- the patient makes a written request that is witnessed, with no pressure, and
- expert panels undertake reports, analyses and reviews.

The Netherlands was the first country in the world to legalise euthanasia in 2002 for those aged 12 years and over. The Act allows for both doctor-administered and patient-administered euthanasia.

Belgium legalised euthanasia later the same year, but only for doctor-administered dying, which can be requested through an advance care directive. In May 2014, Belgium allowed those under the age of 18 access to euthanasia, with additional strict conditions including terminal illness, the ability of the minor to understand what euthanasia means and consent of parents or guardians. The first, and only case to 2017, of child euthanasia was enacted in September 2014 but details are sparse.

Luxembourg legalised doctor-administered and patient-administered euthanasia in 2009.

In the United States there are no Federal laws for euthanasia, which remains illegal in most of the states except Oregon (1994), Washington (2008), Vermont (2013), California (2015), Montana (2015), Colorado (2016) and Washington DC (2017). These states allow patient-administered euthanasia called 'physician-assisted dying'. Doctor-administered euthanasia or any form of assisted suicide outside these medical Acts remains a criminal offence.

Switzerland's 1994 Criminal Code states that assisting suicide is a crime only if undertaken out of self-interested motivations. This legalises patient-administered euthanasia without a specific euthanasia law in place. Doctor-administered euthanasia remains unlawful.

Canada enacted federal legislation in June 2016 to legalise doctor-administered and patient-administered euthanasia called 'medical assistance in dying', with strict conditions, procedures and reporting. The Act disallows advance care directives. After the first six months, of the total 507 medically assisted deaths, only three were patient administered.

Columbia legalised doctor-administered and patient-administered euthanasia in the terminally ill in 2015.

Finland legalised patient-administered euthanasia in end-of-life care in 2012.

Germany legalised patient-administered euthanasia in 2015 on 'an individual basis out of altruistic motives'. Doctor-administered euthanasia and 'commercial suicide businesses' are illegal.

*

Dr Patel's misunderstanding of euthanasia in his presentation, and the passion that can be evoked by the topic, were exemplified at the dinner party the previous month, hosted by my neighbours Mike and Mary. The other invited couple was Bill, a high school teacher, a slight man with big spectacles, and his journalist wife Joan, a petite blonde. The table conversation drifted to an article Joan had recently written in the local community newspaper. It had a long-winded title: '*Why I do not want to lie in a hospital bed Brain Dead for the rest of my life!!!'* with three exclamation marks, essentially her opinion piece in support of euthanasia.

She turned towards me. 'I suppose like all doctors, you are against euthanasia? Did you read it?', she asked me guardedly with an impassive face, but her eyes glinted.

'Yes. The title had caught my attention. I initially thought that your article was about brain death', I said, without wishing to point out that a brain-dead patient does not live, let alone lie indefinitely in a hospital bed. A brain-dead person is not a good *cause célèbre* choice to champion euthanasia; you cannot kill a person who is already dead.

'Same thing! Doctors refusing a patient's requested right to die', she retorted. Her face tightened and she rested her hands on the edge of the table, seemingly ready for battle. The table fell silent. Bill shifted on his chair. Mike looked intently at his plate. Mary's face wrinkled in apprehension. Di, my wife, fixed a polite smile.

I did not wish to ignite an argument. I nodded. 'Usually I'm the one accused of committing euthanasia', I said lamely. Joan unexpectedly laughed, gallantly taking my cue for both of us to back off. Everyone else broke into a smile, a silent group exhalation of relief. The pall of unease lifted from the table. No one wanted a heated debate at that time of night on euthanasia, the mother of all medical controversies.

'Any more shiraz?', Joan asked.

*

Arguments for legalising euthanasia

Debates on euthanasia are impassioned. However, considerations for or against legalising euthanasia should not confuse other mislabelled forms of death – mentioned above – with active voluntary euthanasia. Religious and cultural arguments should be excluded. Arguments on each side can be persuasive but can also have weaknesses. These are arguments supporting legalising euthanasia.

DEATH WITH DIGNITY

A patient may suffer severe pain from terminal illness, and pain relief may not be adequate even with medication doses that may hasten death. If the patient requests euthanasia to end their insufferable pain, it is humanly decent to accede to that wish. The patient can then 'die with dignity'. However, pain is not the primary reason that patients seek euthanasia (see later in this chapter). The majority of deaths caused by euthanasia are patients with cancer, but evidence suggests that patients who requested euthanasia infrequently experience severe pain and, of these, only a minority feared inadequate pain relief. Over the past 15–20 years, pain medicine has been established as a specialty in Australia, and pain specialists today can offer better pain management than other doctors.

RIGHT TO CHOOSE

The right to actively end one's life is a personal one. The principle of patient autonomy is fundamental to common law and one respected by the medical profession. Although autonomy is a central tenet in refusing treatment (a request for *omission* of treatment even if death may be the consequence), its value is different in euthanasia: a request for *an active act* to secure death. The two deaths are different not in degree but in kind. It is possible to respect autonomy without supporting euthanasia. In a democratic society, personal autonomy in each and every circumstance in life cannot apply with no boundary; 'free speech' is an example. It may be a private affair about a patient's right, but it is a public and society-wide issue because it involves the state sanctioning acts to commit death under certain conditions.

TRANSPARENCY

Legalising euthanasia would provide proper regulation and scrutiny to safeguard patients and doctors. Clear, precise laws would provide oversight and rulings by expert bodies. Every case of euthanasia would require a thoughtful and comprehensive approach, with complete attention to consent, underlying disease, suffering, prognosis and other options for care. There would be a strict, inflexible adherence to the law, without exceptions. No one would 'fall through gaps'. However, anti-euthanasia advocates query whether politicians, health authorities and doctors can competently deliver these specific vital elements in *each and every case*.

DYING IS NOT PROLONGED

If the patient is dying with a terminal illness and if the dying process is unbearable, the patient should have the right to reduce this period of suffering. Also, valuable resources of skilled staff, equipment, beds and medications to prolong the life of such a patient who wishes to die can be better channelled to life-saving treatments of other patients. Economic reasoning to support legalising euthanasia is valid but is a two-edged sword (see later in this chapter).

Arguments against legalising euthanasia

The following are arguments against legalising euthanasia; some have weaknesses too.

PALLIATIVE CARE

The World Health Organization defines palliative care as 'an approach that improves the quality of life of patients and their families facing the problem associated with life-threatening illness, through the prevention and relief of suffering by means of early identification and impeccable assessment and treatment of pain and other problems, physical, psycho-social and spiritual.'[4] Palliative care is an established medical specialty in Australia. The quality of palliative care today is much more advanced than over a decade ago when euthanasia was first legalised in the Netherlands. Palliative care specialists work in multidisciplinary healthcare teams to provide the best-quality end-of-life care in the face of death until natural death occurs, whereas euthanasia's intent is a sudden death, by a single active intervention, only minutes in duration.

The primary reason most often reported for patients seeking euthanasia was psychological suffering such as depression, hopelessness and loss of autonomy and dignity, and not pain, contrary to the expectations of the public.[5] In Belgium, psychiatric patients who made the most requests for euthanasia suffered not from pain, but from psychological disorders.[6] Palliative care, with attention to pain and symptom control and psychological, emotional and social support, is thus valuable in terminal illness. With effective palliative care, the terminally ill can die with equal or more dignity than euthanasia will provide. Its option should not be underplayed in the quest for euthanasia. Indeed, in jurisdictions where euthanasia is legal, reports indicate that some patients who received euthanasia were not enrolled in palliative care.[3] Euthanasia is not a panacea in end-of-life care or even a substitute for palliative care. It is a disproportionate response to problems of end-of-life care that needs more care and money. True, unfortunately not every patient with terminal illness has access to good palliative care, and governments should first address this issue.

SLIPPERY SLOPE

This 'slippery slope' argument reasons that, in removing legal barriers to euthanasia, society would then accept increasing motivations of actively terminating life and with fewer checks. The core argument for euthanasia is that it offers a compassionate, peaceful last journey for those with a terminal illness and unbearable suffering. However, once it becomes an acceptable medical practice ('normalisation'), requests for euthanasia would grow. The increase in supplicants could extend to those *with no elements of terminal illness and/or intractable suffering.* In Belgium, deaths by euthanasia rose from 235 in 2003 to 2012 by 2015, in the Netherlands from 2331 in 2008 to 5516 in 2015 and in Switzerland from 50 in 1998 to 836 in 2014, with compound annual growth rates of 19.6%, 13.1% and 19.2% respectively.[7] Increases are also seen in Oregon and Quebec. Two years after legalising euthanasia for adults, Belgium extended euthanasia to *anyone.* Anti-euthanasia supporters ask how lawmakers could expect a minor to understand the meaning of euthanasia, as decreed in Belgium's law. When active termination of life becomes a choice for competent people, could the line that excludes incompetent people from euthanasia eventually blur? Could euthanasia even become acceptable for people with disabilities? Hitler's euthanasia record is an unhelpful, over-the-top example of the 'slippery slope' argument against euthanasia, but the risk of a chain of related events that may culminate in negative effects for the community is valid. In Europe, from initially being limited to people in terminal illness *and* intolerable pain, euthanasia in the Netherlands has expanded to include old people and, in Belgium, people suffering from depression. The media has reported requests for euthanasia by people who have no terminal illness or suffering but are just 'tired of life'. Other sick or disabled people, thinking of their families, might feel obliged to offer up their deaths. Hence, can safeguards be guaranteed to avert vulnerable people from succumbing to an 'easy exit', or unscrupulous people from exploiting the euthanasia process for gain?

Despite a progressive ('creeping') increase in euthanasia deaths from evidence mentioned earlier, the numbers are still relatively small after 'normalisation' in euthanasia-legal countries, at 0.3%–4.6% of all reported deaths. Some cases though were, and may still be, unreported as the participating doctors and nurses did not perceive them as euthanasia, because the patients were close to death.[8] Nonetheless, there is no suggestion of widespread abuse (not all requests are granted) and no evidence in any jurisdiction that vulnerable patients have received euthanasia without their request.[3]

BAD DEATH, GOOD DEATH

With capital punishment, convicted murderers or criminals are executed. Australia, like many countries, has abolished the death penalty because society considers it inhumane and immoral. Also, an executed prisoner may be proven innocent years later, with better 'cold case' investigation techniques. Euthanasia ends the life of a patient, albeit at the patient's request. Both are technically state-sanctioned killings. It would seem paradoxical today for society to view the execution of prisoners as an uncivilised 'bad death' and yet euthanasia as an appropriate 'good death'. Similarly, society laments the deaths of its people by suicide, particularly the young. Australia's suicide rate is considered in crisis, with 2866 suicides (11.8 per 100,000 or 7.85 deaths each day) in 2017. Legalising euthanasia by assisted suicide would seem inconsistent with public health efforts to address the social and mental distresses that drive suicidal deaths, sending a confusing message to desperate adults and confused teenagers.

It is a common belief that euthanasia is a painless and flawless process, but such a 'good death' is not always realistic or good.[9] A study in the Netherlands reported that 5.5% of all cases of euthanasia had a technical problem; 3.7% had a complication (including nausea, vomiting and muscle spasms), 6.9% had problems with completing euthanasia and 1.1% of patients did not die but awoke from coma.[10] These are not *euthanatos* or 'easy deaths'.

*

'Medical ward 3 will take Mrs Rebold. I'll discharge her', Rosemary Smith told me. Mary Rebold was a 59-year-old school teacher who had been admitted unconscious three days previously from an overdose of antidepressants. Intentional, self-inflicted drug overdoses were common in the 1970s and 1980s, making up 10% of non-surgical admissions to ICU. Presentations to hospital could be predicted around Easter, Christmas, New Year's Day and long weekend holidays, perhaps when vulnerable people felt depressed because they could see others being happy and they were not. With improved mental healthcare services and mandatory packaging of dangerous drug tablets in aluminium foil (instead of bulk pills in containers), the incidence of drug overdose dropped. One's enthusiasm to gulp down tablets would tend to waiver after breaking the individual foil of the tenth tablet. Today, Mary Rebold's admission was uncommon, and she responded well to treatment – mechanical ventilation and drugs to counter low blood pressure and abnormal heart rhythms.

Suicide is today no longer a criminal offence in many countries. We had spent valuable resources to save the life of a person who wanted to kill herself. If she had succeeded, her death would have been viewed as a 'bad death', sad and 'without dignity'. If she were in a parallel universe that endorsed patient-administered euthanasia, valuable resources from the same healthcare pool would be used to end her life, just as she wished. Her death would then be viewed as a celebratory 'good death', and a death 'with dignity'. Such a parallel universe exists today in countries that accept patient-assisted euthanasia under varying conditions.

*

ECONOMICS

Government cutbacks in healthcare spending pose a threat to those who are medically and economically marginalised. Inadequate funding for palliative care means that many cannot access its services. Opponents of euthanasia claim that the demand for euthanasia could be eliminated, or at least reduced, with high-quality palliative and nursing care available across society. As the ageing population grows, health providers – government or private health insurers – may come under pressure to look at euthanasia as a means of cost containment. Major illness can obviously drain family finances, and with legalised euthanasia the sick will also be under pressure to choose a cheaper care alternative; euthanasia may be seen as a 'duty to die' choice. Chronically ill elderly parents may also be pressurised to 'move on', to cease being a burden and erode inheritances. However, evidence of these scenarios of economics impinging on decisions for euthanasia has not been demonstrated. Finally, legalised euthanasia for some will need resources for implementation – valuable resources that should be better utilised to provide quality palliative care for all.

Ethical and moral issues in medicine

Legalisation of euthanasia gives rise to other issues for the medical profession and society. What is the right answer to each of these below?

DO NOT KILL

'Do not kill' has been a core ethical principle of every civilisation. The Hippocratic Oath from the 4th century BCE, which serves as a professional contract for doctors to uphold ethical standards, has a promise to 'first do no harm' when caring for patients. In 1948, the World Medical Association adopted this vow as the *Declaration of Geneva*.[11] The United Nations General Assembly adopted the *Universal Declaration of Human Rights*[12] in 1948 to espouse that '*Everyone has the right to life.*' All these affirmations have an underlying ethos that human life must be respected and preserved, with which euthanasia would not be compatible. Hence most doctors and medical bodies oppose euthanasia.

WHO PULLS THE TRIGGER?

The objectives of medicine are to cure, to care, to alleviate suffering and to do no harm (non-maleficence). In euthanasia, the doctor has a direct role to effect the death of the patient, albeit with good intentions. However, to the medical profession, this motive conflicts with our code to do no harm. Medical ethics recognise the right of a doctor to reject the practice of euthanasia even if it is in accordance with the law. Who will then 'pull the trigger' – that is, be charged with the responsibility for enacting euthanasia? In Switzerland and Germany, euthanasia can operate outside of established medicine. What training, supervision, scrutiny and reporting of practice would be required for euthanasia practition-ers? How would practical euthanasia be taught to students of healthcare professions?

DOCTOR–PATIENT RELATIONSHIP

One of the fears of legislated euthanasia is that it will undermine the doctor–patient relationship, destroying the trust and confidence traditionally built in such a relationship. Casting doctors in the role of euthanasia practitioners could challenge and compromise the objectives of medicine as a profession. Can you still trust your doctor who has recently become a specialist in euthanasia? Another fear is that the practice of euthanasia could corrupt the character of doctors, if economics and healthcare rationing begin to influence who can live and who must die.

What of the future?

It is possible that, with sociological changes worldwide, more countries will legalise euthanasia in the future. Then will euthanasia change the landscape of aged care? How will vulnerable people be protected from slipping through 'cracks in the floor'? How do we keep profiteers in check? Will there be mental health consequences in families and health professionals? Relatives who witnessed the death by euthanasia of a loved one are reported to have a higher incidence of posttraumatic stress disorder (PTSD) and depression than the general population in the Netherlands.[10] The same disorder may afflict the healthcare team.[13]

⋆

The Chair of the peer review meeting rotated each month between the heads of departments. Dr Alistair Shadrick, head of orthopaedics, was the Chair at the meeting of Dr Patel's presentation. He was a burly, massive 55-year-old with hands like spades who had played prop forward for Sydney University's rugby union team. A favourite specialist of sporting organisations, he did not suffer fools gladly. Dr Shadrick leaned forward, towering over the table and lowered his head, his bushy eyebrows furrowed. He did not look happy.

'Even a dumb bastard like me knows that the prognosis of a ruptured aortic aneurysm in a moribund elderly patient with heart disease is zero, nil, zilch!', he said. 'She would have died on the way to theatre or on the operating table. It would have been a further waste of Red Cross blood, theatre use and time of all staff. Worse of all, she would have been put through unnecessary suffering. Calling that euthanasia is nonsense. Sit down please, Dr Patel. Next case!', he bellowed.

*

Reflections

- The concept of euthanasia, bringing a 'good death' to someone with a terminal illness and in insufferable pain, is complex in real-life medical practice.
- Non-voluntary euthanasia is never acceptable.
- Some euthanasia advocates do not consider terminal illness and insufferable pain preconditions as vital elements for euthanasia. Euthanasia practice in some jurisdictions has included subjects without terminal illness or insufferable pain.
- Many support euthanasia because they confuse non-euthanasia deaths as 'euthanasia' and wish such dying be legally permitted to proceed. They are in modern medical practice.
- Arguments for and against euthanasia have holes.
- Safeguards cannot always be guaranteed.
- Allowing doctor-administered and patient-assisted euthanasia, but banning the death penalty and deterring suicides, are conflicting and confusing moral paths.
- Good palliative care should always be the principal approach. Tread your own path, but best don't go there.

References

1. Lawrence DH. The ship of death. In: Abrams MH, editor. *The Norton anthology of English literature*, vol. 2. 6th ed. New York: Norton; 1993. p. 2128.
2. Binding K, Hoche A. *The release of the destruction of life devoid of value*. Leipzig, Germany: Felix Meiner; 1920. reprinted in paperback 1975 by RL Sassone, Santa Ana, CA.
3. Materstvedt LJ, Clark D, Ellershaw J, Førde R, Gravgaard AM, Müller-Busch HC, et al; EAPC Ethics Task Force. Euthanasia and physician-assisted suicide: a view from an EAPC ethics task force. *Palliat Med* 2003;17:97–101, discussion 102–79.
4. World Health Organization. *WHO definition of palliative care*. Geneva: WHO; n.d. www.who.int/cancer/palliative/definition/en.
5. Emanuel EJ, Onwuteaka-Philipsen BD, Urwin JW, Cohen J. Attitudes and practices of euthanasia and physician-assisted suicide in the United States, Canada, and Europe. *JAMA* 2016;316(1):79–90.

6. Thienpont L, Verhofstadt M, Van Loon T, Distelmans W, Audenaert K, De Deyn PP. Euthanasia requests, procedures and outcomes for 100 Belgian patients suffering from psychiatric disorders. *BMJ Open* 2015;5(7):e007454.

7. Mulino D. *MLC Minority report. Inquiry into end of life choices.* Melbourne, VIC: Parliament of Victoria; 2016.

8. Smets T, Bilsen J, Cohen J, Rurup ML, Mortier F, Deliens L. Reporting of euthanasia in medical practice in Flanders, Belgium: cross sectional analysis of reported and unreported cases. *BMJ* 2010;341:c5174.

9. Emanuel E. Euthanasia and physician-assisted suicide: focus on the data. *Med J Aust* 2017;206(8):339–40.

10. Groenewoud JH, van der Heide A, Onwuteaka-Philipsen BD, Willems DL, van der Maas PJ, van der Wal G. Clinical problems with the performance of euthanasia and physician-assisted suicide in the Netherlands. *N Engl J Med* 2000;342(8):551–6.

11. World Medical Association. *Declaration of Geneva.* Geneva: WMA; 1948. https://www.wma.net/.

12. United Nations. *Universal declaration of human rights.* Geneva: WHO; 1948. www.un.org/en/universal-declaration-human-rights/index.html.

13. Van Marwijk H, Haverkate I, van Royen P, The AM. Impact of euthanasia on primary care physicians in The Netherlands. *Palliat Med* 2007;21(7):609–14.

11

Organ donation

The greatest gift there is to offer

How far that little candle throws his beams!
So shines a good deed in a weary world.

William Shakespeare (1564–1616) in the *Merchant of Venice*
(about 1596)

*

A necessary component of end-of-life care is discussing organ donation with the family of a potential organ donor. It is a duty of organ donation specialists or ICU doctors to engage in this *family donation conversation* after confirmation of brain death or before the heartbeat stops. Care of organ donors is an important and frequent assignment in end-of-life care in the ICU.

*

This was a continuation of the conversation we all dread. 'Sheila, we talked two hours ago that we had tested Bill and he is brain dead. He will never recover and he is legally dead', I said.

Sheila nodded, holding back her tears. She was the young wife of Bill Watson, a 24-year-old motorcyclist who had been hit by a truck four days previously. He had sustained massive head, abdominal and skeletal injuries.

'I am sorry', I continued, 'but I have a duty to raise with you the question of organ donation. Sheila, did you know that Bill had registered as an organ donor? But we will proceed with his wish only if you consent.'

Sheila burst out crying, not able to hold herself back any longer. Maisie and Dick, her parents, jumped out of their chairs to comfort her, claiming her three-month-old infant from her shaking arms. Helen, Bill's bed nurse, stood by looking and feeling utterly wretched.

After they had composed themselves, I explained further the process and the preciousness of the gift of organ donation. 'Have you any questions?', I asked.

Sheila shook her head, her face lost in paper tissues. She settled after a while and then looked up, with red eyes. 'Yes', she said softly, holding her baby close. 'We had discussed this. He would want this.' Her distraught parents put their arms around her.

*

Organ and tissue donation

In Australia, the Organ and Tissue Authority (OTA), with its DonateLife agencies in each state and territory, oversees organ donation and transplantation. Organ and tissue donation involves removing organs and tissues from a person who has died (a donor) and transplanting them into someone who is very ill or dying (a recipient). Organ transplantation can save and significantly improve the lives of many people, and is the only hope for a healthy life for those with organ failure. In Australia in 2017, requests were made to 1093 families of potential donors, with a 59% consent rate. Some cases did not proceed because of various medical reasons, and 510 deceased organ donors – a *conversion rate* of 79% – saved and transformed the lives of 1402 Australian recipients. In addition, 273 living donors helped the same number of recipients. Nonetheless, at any time there are about 1400 people in Australia on the waiting list for organ transplants.

Most organ donations are cadaveric, 75% following brain death (i.e. donation after brain death, DBD) and a quarter after the heartbeat stops (i.e. donation after circulatory death, DCD). Living organ donors number about half that of cadaveric donors. A living donor is someone who donates a kidney or partial liver to another person, usually a relative or close friend, who has end-stage disease. Organs that can be transplanted include the heart, lungs, liver, kidneys, intestine and pancreas. Tissues that can be transplanted include heart valves and other heart tissue, bone, tendons, ligaments, skin and parts of the eye, such as the cornea and sclera. Only a few medical conditions preclude donation of organs. The condition of donated organs and tissues and how a donor dies are important (i.e. within organ-viable timeframes for retrieval and transplantation). Older Australians can be donors, with no definitive age limit. One donor can transform the lives of 10 or more people.

Australia ranks 17th in the world for organ donation, with 20.7 donors per million population (DPMP) in 2016. Spain, at 43.8 DPMP, has been the consistent world leader, followed by Croatia and Portugal, at 39.5 DPMP and 32.7 DPMP respectively (all three, interestingly, being predominantly Catholic countries). Spain's high performance donation rate is attributable to an excellent nationwide infrastructure, high ratios of ICU beds and acceptance by their people of organ donation as an end-of-life event.

*

She glared at me with narrowed, steely eyes and flared nostrils. 'He wants to donate his organs but you are not taking them!', Mrs Cathy Blewett said empathically. She was the fortyish-aged daughter of Joe Costello, the 76-year-old in bed 16, who had been admitted three days previously following a heart attack at home. While in the emergency department, he had suffered a cardiac arrest but was resuscitated and admitted to ICU. However, his condition deteriorated quickly with his end-stage heart failure, and we did not expect him to survive. I had just communicated the bad news to the family before her astonishing outburst.

'We don't know if your father registered for organ donation', I said. 'We did not check the national organ donation register because he is an unsuitable donor owing to his age and illness. At any rate, we would first need your family's consent, but we do not want your father's organs', I tried to reassure her. Her elderly mother sat next to her, dressed in black. She clutched her handbag but remained silent, her eyes misted in grief and confusion. Cathy's burly husband in a fluorescent yellow 'hi-viz' shirt with shorts and boots – the tradesman's uniform – sat on her other side, leaning forward with hands clasped, unsure of what to say or do.

'You doctors take organs without permission. Over 80% of men over 70 years old who die have their organs removed without anyone knowing', Cathy continued, belligerent in her misguided concern for her father.

'Cathy, I don't know where you got your information from, but it is incorrect. We don't target elderly dead men for organs. Also, consent from the patient or family for all procedures is paramount in our work. What would we want with dead organs?'

'For *science*!', she retorted, glaring with pursed lips at her perceived organ plunderer.

'I promise you, Cathy, we will not do that. May I suggest that you spend time with Mr Costello at his bedside?' I ended the conversation.

Cathy's statements simply dumbfounded me. She believed that, today, we could practise body or organ snatching like gravediggers in Victorian London. Much injudicious fear surrounds subjects like organ donation and brain death, but her views were gold standard for obtuse ignorance. The nurses told me later that she harboured other such unconventional views. Apparently she was also an 'anti-vaxxer', stridently opposed to vaccinating her kids, with opinions gleaned from gossip among her peer group of mothers.

*

Consent

The Australian Organ Donation Register is a national register for people over 16 years old to voluntarily register their wish to be an organ donor after death. In 2017, only 34% of eligible Australians were registered. Regardless of wishes as registered, consent is still required from the family for doctors to proceed to organ retrieval. Registration is important, as 90% of families of those registered consent to donation, and only 44% if there is no registration or known choice.

A number of OECD countries have *presumed-consent* laws on organ donation. This is a default 'yes' option of organ donation if the individual does not make a premortem choice to 'opt-out' of donating organs. Few countries follow an absolutist rule, with many adopting various shades of a family veto. Some studies have attributed increases in organ donation to varied reasons, including presumed-consent laws.[1] Along with New Zealand, the US, the UK and Canada, Australia practises informed consent that requires a final family consent. Viewed thus it is not a state mandate, but rather the family's affirmative choice to donate organs, which can help them derive something positive out of a tragedy. Simply changing the law to presumed consent (of any shade) will not necessarily result in significant increases in organ donation rate, as there are many interrelating determinants.

Refusal of organ donation

Families refuse consent often for the same reasons – for example, the patient has suffered enough, they do not know what he / she would want, fear of disfigurement from surgery, extra costs and delaying the funeral and burial process. They should be reassured that these presumptions are incorrect. Some family members may disagree for personal reasons or are dissatisfied with the healthcare process. Organ donation or procurement for money is a criminal offence in Australia.

Donation after brain death (DBD)

DBD is the most common (75%) of cadaveric donations. Once brain death has been confirmed, consent obtained and necessary tests and arrangements completed, the patient is moved to the operating theatre. Medications and ventilation are continued, but ceased during organ retrieval surgery. This pathway of 'beating-heart' donation by a legally dead person offers the best viability of organs. Whether or not donation proceeds, care, dignity and respect for the family's wishes are always maintained during this end-of-life care.

Donation after circulatory death (DCD)

A quarter of cadaveric donations are via DCD. This pathway was introduced in recent years to increase organ donation rates. If continuing treatment is futile and not in the patient's best interests, the doctors will discuss withdrawing life-sustaining treatment with the family and, if the patient is a suitable donor, organ donation by DCD as well. Treatment is withdrawn, and death is diagnosed when breathing and the heartbeat stop (by absence of a palpable or monitored pulse). After a mandatory observation period of five minutes to confirm absence of the heartbeat, death is declared and organ donation proceeds. The dead person is then moved quickly to the operating theatre. Obviously the viability of organs depends on the timeframe of absent or poor circulatory perfusion by a dying heart. The procedure is abandoned if death does not occur after 90 minutes (or at any time, should the family change their decision). Once again, care, dignity and respect for the family's wishes are maintained even if donation does not proceed.

Organ retrieval surgery

Surgery is arranged after having confirmed with the family which organs and tissues they agreed to be donated. Similar to any operation, a surgical incision is made in order to retrieve the organs. This wound is later closed and covered with a dressing; the surgery does not result in any disfigurement. Retrieved organs are then transported to another operating theatre or hospital where transplantation will take place. The family members may then view the deceased if they wish. They will face no costs and the procedure will not affect funeral arrangements unless required by a coroner's investigation. DonateLife agencies provide access to bereavement support and care.

Organ transplantation

Transplant teams determine the allocation of retrieved organs and tissue according to national protocols. These are based on a number of criteria, including the most urgent need, the best match and waiting lists, to ensure the best possible outcome of the donation. In Australia, if there is no local suitable recipient, the specific organ is allocated to the next rostered state or territory or New Zealand. By law, the identities of donors and recipients are kept anonymous, but donor families and transplant recipients can communicate (without identification) through DonateLife.

Religions

The major religions are generally supportive of organ donation (Chapter 12 Religions at the end of life), but there are individual uncertainties in the interpretation of certain laws and beliefs. Examples of potential obstacles to organ donation are in defining death, interpretations of teachings, and religious rituals and observances. Racial and ethnic communities may have beliefs apart from religious ones that are unclear about donating organs. An example is the commitment for the deceased's body to remain intact and unviolated in death. Empathetic discussions involving hospital's particular religious or ethnic official will help.

*

Some weeks later, Sheila Watson paid an unexpected visit to the ICU bringing her son – now an active 5-month-old – and accompanied by her parents Maisie and Dick. She looked composed, settled and healthy. They thanked us for the care of Bill. DonateLife had contacted her, she told us. Bill's lungs went to a local recipient, his kidneys to two recipients, and his liver and lungs went interstate. The organs had saved and improved the lives of five people, plus more from his donated tissues. Her decision to respect Bill's wish had provided her with strength and purpose to cope with his death, and to live for their son. She felt that he had not died in vain.

*

Reflections

- The organ donation family conversation is an important component of end-of-life care.
- Organ donation can be viewed as an opportunity to save lives and improve the quality of life for many people.
- Everyone is encouraged to discuss with their family their wish for organ donation.
- Everyone is encouraged to register in the Australian Organ Donation Register.

References

1. Shepard L, O'Carroll RE, Ferguson E. An international comparison of deceased and living organ donation / transplant rates in opt-in and opt-out systems: a panel study. *BMC Med* 2014;12:131.

PART V

Faiths

Religions at the end of life

Walking home with God

A man's ethical behaviour should be based effectually on sympathy, education, and social ties – no religious basis is necessary. Man would indeed be in a poor way if he had to be restrained by fear of punishment and hope of reward after death.

Albert Einstein (1879–1955), German born scientist who developed the Theory of Relativity.

A man can die but once; we owe God a death.

William Shakespeare (1564–1616), *Henry IV* Part II, Act III, Scene 2

*

For some people with a terminal illness, having a religious faith helps in coping with their emotions. Religious factors can influence patients' and families' decisions at the end of life. They may have preferences in end-of-life care and care after immediate death. Awareness of these religious needs when communicating with patients and families are thus important in end-of-life care. Doctors, nurses and carers need to understand the basic tenets of the major world religions. Treatment plans that respect religious wishes will show regard for families and reduce their stress.

*

Mike, my neighbour, appeared in my backyard to return the pair of shears that he had borrowed. 'Thanks for this Tom. Reckon they'll need this to cut off Father Nedd's balls?', he said, referring to the main news item of the day – that of the Anglican priest David Nedd's trial for abusing two boys. 'Never ending, these paedophilia cases. Wonder what they teach them in theology schools? This time it's an Anglican, not a Catholic. No wonder nana was such an atheist', he said, referring to his late grandmother. 'She was born a Catholic, you know, but she brought up her four boys as atheists. So dad's anti-religion; mum has issues with that sometimes.' He paused. His eyes looked down in reflection. 'Interesting point though', he continued. 'When nana was dying, dad didn't want to raise her last rites with the ICU nurses, but mum wanted to. No one offered anyway. I know you're not religious, Tom. I reckon you're safe in your work. The ICU is free from religions', he concluded, smiling, pleased with his powers of deduction. He handed over the shears. I noticed that he hadn't cleaned them.

'Not exactly, Mike', I said, taking the dirty shears off him. 'I'll tell you all about religions and us doctors. Want a beer?'

*

In a modern secular society such as Australia, religion does not dictate how medicine is practised in public institutions. Different religions have their views on death and the care for the dying, some of which may not align with present understandings of medicine or with specific hospital protocols. The importance of religion differs between individuals. Cultures, political views and life's events also influence choices and behaviours; thoughts of family members in the context of health dilemmas cannot always be predicted. Nonetheless, in times of crises, people may be guided by the religious perspectives that they know and from which they can draw comfort. In the face of death, religions have provided mechanisms for coping with all the areas of life affected by the death of a loved one. Hence, religious beliefs may influence decisions made by patients, their families and their doctors.[1,2]

Family communications on end-of-life care, futile treatment and withdrawal of life support need to consider religious beliefs and cultural values. The main religions have a commonality of basic values – the sanctity of life and the dignity of the patient

– but understanding the views of different religions will facilitate staff to discuss, and even negotiate, treatment with families. Conversations with the family can explore interpretations of dilemmas, degrees of differences from traditional religion, cut-and-dry rulings and moral concepts. They may also reveal erroneous assumptions by the lay professional staff. The main areas where religions may conflict with contemporary medical care are accepting brain death as death, organ donation, withdrawal of treatment and futile life support.[3,4] Some writings by religious scholars and officers on the concept and pathophysiology of brain death unfortunately do not reflect modern medical practice, often labelling coma and vegetative states as brain death (Chapter 9 Brain death and vegetative states).

Religions with Western traditions have perceptions of *personhood*, where an individual is a finite human being, with characteristics and feelings, and alive from birth to death. In Eastern religious traditions, personhood is not defined in physical terms, and indigenous traditions appreciably influence ideas, such as death being a process that continues after the body has been declared dead by lay doctors. Western religions do not agree on precisely how to determine death, but they are able to locate a moment of death in the body. In Eastern religions, the cessation of heart and brain function is not the end of dying, but rather the beginning of the process of death and rebirth. The main religions in the world will be presented in the following sections to see how they may influence end-of-life decisions in acute hospital wards.

Judaism[5]

There about 15 million people in the world who are Jewish. Judaism has a variety of movements, the three largest being Orthodox Judaism, Conservative Judaism and Reform Judaism. They differ mainly in their approaches to Jewish law and the authority of the rabbis. Orthodox Judaism maintains that the Torah (the first part of the Jewish bible) and Jewish law are divine and should be strictly followed. Reform Judaism is more liberal, with Conservative Judaism being 'in-between' traditional. Special religious courts historically enforced Jewish law, but the practice of Judaism today is mostly voluntary. There is no single central authority, and responses to moral issues depend on rabbis and scholars who interpret the sacred texts, and on cultural considerations. Views differ between movements, but the central tenet of Jewish law and tradition is the sanctity of human life. To preserve life is a duty that overrides self-determination; to actively shorten life (including by suicide and euthanasia) is prohibited. Jewish law also recognises a duty to alleviate suffering. In modern times, to exercise autonomy in refusing life-saving treatment raises questions. This may be permissible when the treatment carries an element of risk to the patient or, if enforced, will cause the patient considerable distress; some oppose this view. The concept of brain death as death is supported by Reform and Conservative Judaism, but not by all followers of Orthodox Judaism. Nonetheless, the assertion that any and all measures must be undertaken to extend life is a minority opinion.

Modern medicine does not differentiate between withdrawing a treatment and withholding a treatment, but in Judaism some argue that withdrawing treatment is tantamount to actively hastening death. However, if a treatment needs to be re-administered, withholding the next course would be permissible. Many authorities have permitted withdrawing treatment in the terminally ill, but only if that did not lead to *immediate death* (which is undefined but would otherwise constitute active hastening of death). Withdrawing life support ventilation is particularly challenging. Death would follow almost immediately, making that option not permissible, but this view is not unanimous. Withdrawing futile life support ventilation can be considered as allowing natural death to occur.

Catholicism[3]

There are about 2.3 billion Christians, or 32% of the world's population of 7.5 billion (as of 2015). Half the Christians are Roman Catholics. The Roman Catholic Church, unlike Judaism, developed a hierarchical structure in its first centuries. Pronouncements on moral issues come from the top, the Papacy or office of the Pope, leader of the Catholic Church. These are based more on biblical moral concepts and they significantly influence the Catholic laity. Statements from Pope Pius XII (1939–58 Papacy) were used to affirm the Catholic position that brain death, as determined by the medical profession, was an appropriate definition of death. Pope John Paul II (1978–2005 Papacy) reaffirmed this view, which is opposed by a few Catholics influenced by wrong interpretations of brain death, such as mistaking coma and persistent vegetative states for brain death. Withdrawing ventilation after the diagnosis of brain death thus presents no difficulties to Catholics.

Catholic teaching accepts the limits of medical technology, based on the ethical reasonings of two theologians: Thomas Aquinas, a 13th-century Italian, and Francisco De Vitoria, a 16th-century Spaniard. Aquinas' schema, called *natural law*, gave rise to the *doctrine of double effect* (Chapter 2 Ethics in death and dying). This ethical principle permits an act for a beneficial effect that may also cause an unintended, bad effect. Doses of opioids for pain relief, for example, may suppress breathing and thus hasten death. The doctrine is acceptable if the act arises from good will, the bad effect is not the means to achieve the good and the effects are proportionately more good than bad. De Vitoria proposed that, to prolong life in the face of imminent death, '*ordinary*' means of treatment are required but '*extraordinary*' means that are burdensome to the patient may be discontinued. Pope John Paul II reiterated these values in 1980, using the terms '*proportionate*' and '*disproportionate*' means. Hence, continuing ventilation in a patient when death is imminent is a 'disproportionate' treatment, and withdrawing ventilation is permissible. Death, which follows, is considered an indirect effect.

Catholic ethics aim to avoid the two extremes: an unrealistic and burdensome prolongation of life when death is imminent (which does not contribute to the overall wellbeing of the patient) and a too-ready acquiescence to withdraw life support because of misplaced compassion or pragmatism that leans towards a disregard for the value of life. Finally, if a Catholic patient is near death, the family may urgently request for a Catholic priest to offer '*Last Rites*' or '*Sacrament of the Sick*', to prepare the dying person's soul for death.

Protestantism[3]

There about 900 million people in the world (37% of all Christians) who are Protestant Christians. Protestantism is a form of Christianity that originated in Germany in 1517 with the Reformation – a movement led by Martin Luther, a theologian and monk, against what he considered as errors in the Roman Catholic Church. The

Reformation then spread in Europe and to the Baltic States. England's King Henry VIII started Anglican Protestantism (the English Reformation) in 1529 because of personal and political motivations rather than a religious dispute. Presbyterian Protestantism originated in Scotland. The main principles of the Reformation were: the *priesthood of believers* that opposes a hierarchical structure, and instead regards believers as 'priests' to participate in affairs of the church, and *Sola Scriptura*, that Scripture alone is authoritative for faith and practice – the Bible is complete, authoritative and true. The Anglican Church also places value on tradition, more like Catholicism. Over the past three centuries, the spread of Protestantism all over the world has spawned various movements, then branches or denominations, the major ones being Lutheran, Anglican, Presbyterian, Methodist, Baptist, Adventist and Pentecostal. Evangelicalism is a movement largely in North America that stresses the preaching of the Gospel, personal conversion ('born again') experiences and active personal commitments to Christ. Today, Protestantism generally refers to Christian denominations other than that of the Catholic or Eastern Orthodox Church.

The numerous Protestant branches and denominations have varying differences in worship (e.g. ordination of women to ministerial or priestly office), and many do not have official statements on criteria to determine death. However, Protestantism in general supports neurological criteria to define brain death, and thus death. The Protestant churches also support the individual's right to make decisions on their care, which can include refusing life support and withdrawing ventilation. On caring for the terminally ill, the churches view relieving suffering as a goal that should not be prevented by technology to prolong dying, especially if suffering is increased.

Eastern Orthodox Christianity[6]

There about 300 million people in the world who are Orthodox Christians, 13% of all Christians. In CE 1054, Medieval Christianity split into two branches: Eastern Orthodox Catholics and Roman Catholics, a separation known as the East–West Schism or Great Schism. Various factors for the Schism had been building up since CE 800, because of the east–west geography of the Roman Empire, language (Latin in the west and Greek in the east), theologies and politics. Eastern Orthodox Catholicism today has followers mainly in the eastern Mediterranean, Asia Minor, Russia and the Balkans. As the capital of the eastern Roman Empire was Byzantine, this branch of Christianity is sometimes called 'Byzantine Christianity'. The churches are self-governing, each with its own geographical (rather than national) title that usually reflects the cultural traditions of its believers. Eastern Orthodox Christianity does not recognise the Pope as the supreme authority over all Christendom, or accept Roman Catholic traditions that developed after the Schism. The nominal head of the Eastern Orthodox Churches is the Patriarch of Constantinople, but he has no real authority over Churches other than his own. Eastern Orthodox Christianity still shares the conviction for basing morality on the Bible. Cultural influences and priestly rituals (with veneration of icons and spiritual meditative prayers) characterise Eastern Orthodox Christianity, whereas Western Christianity's viewpoint is guided more by a practical and legal mentality.

Similar to all religions, life is valued as being sacred, and euthanasia and suicide are forbidden. However, statements on end-of-life issues are few, and in many independent Eastern Orthodox churches (e.g. Greek, Russian, Serbian, Romanian, Bulgarian, Coptic and Orthodox Church in America) views on certain issues vary. Acceptance of brain death, organ donation and withdrawing futile treatment can be unclear, confusing and not universal. Transplantation of animal parts, such as pig heart valves, is universally unacceptable. The Greek Orthodox Church has hesitations on recognising brain death, but allows termination of ventilator therapy in a brain-dead patient to proceed to organ donation. To the Church of Romania, however, donating an organ is tantamount to committing suicide, even if it is done to save another's life (and the donor has already been declared dead). All Orthodox churches, as a principle, reject intentional shortening of life and, in general, do not allow the withholding and withdrawing of treatment, except when death is imminent. Tube feeding cannot be withheld or withdrawn, regardless of the prognosis of recovery.

*

'They all wore burqas', Jane Asquith said in the staff room. She was referring to the family of Mr Mohamad bin Razak, her patient in bed 15, an elderly Muslim man from Malaysia. He had been visiting his two sons and their families now living in Australia when he contracted pneumonia. Being a chronic heavy smoker, he developed respiratory failure that warranted admission to ICU for ventilation. He had a large family, and the ICU receptionist often had to exercise amateur crowd control in the occupancy of the visitors' waiting room.

'All the women wore them, even the girls. Why wear them here? We're not used to these Eastern religions', Jane concluded, her face pinched in perplexed exasperation.

'Actually, they're wearing hijabs, a headscarf covering hair and neck but not the face. Burqas are veils covering the entire body and face, with a mesh across the eyes. They're simply following their religious beliefs. The Koran calls for women to be covered and be modest. The reference to dress and covering the head is open to interpretations that have been shaped by centuries of cultures in different nations. And Islam is a *Western* tradition religion, not Eastern, because with Judaism and Christianity they trace their roots to a single ancestor, Abraham', I informed her. She had not intended to be offensive; just simply expressing her lack of knowledge of Islam and, like many people in Western societies, of the other main 'non-Western' religions – Buddhism and Hinduism.

*

Islam[7]

There are about 1.8 billion people in the world who are Muslims, 23% of the world population. They share with Judaism and Christianity the ancestor Abraham and the way they construe human life: the individual is a creation of God, or Allah, and the person's life begins at a specific time and their death is determined by the cessation of body organs such as the heart, lungs or brain. As a religion since the 7th century based on the visions of the prophet Mohammad, its sources of moral authority are the *Koran* (the holy text), the *Sunnah* (sayings and deeds of the prophet), the consensus of scholars and interpretations of other appropriate authorities. Interpretations can vary, as there is no single person or body vested with the final assertion.

The framework of Muslim life is the *Five Pillars of Islam*: the testimony of faith, prayer, giving support to the needy, fasting during the month of Ramadan, and the pilgrimage to Mecca once in a lifetime. Islam split into two denominations after the death of the prophet Mohammad, because of a dispute about his successor. Shia Islam (predominant in Iran) has a formal clergy and a hierarchy of spiritual leadership up to the Supreme Imam, whereas Sunnis (predominant in Saudi Arabia) have no formal clergy but have scholars and jurists instead.

Islam has deep respect for science and medicine, and Muslim doctors have been influential in developing approaches in bioethical issues. According to Islam, life is a precious gift bestowed by Allah and death is seen as something predestined by Allah, but Islamic texts do not precisely define death or the criteria for declaring death. The First International Conference on Islamic Medicine in Kuwait in 1981 endorsed an Islamic Code of Medical Ethics. The Kuwait document declares that doctors should not transgress their limitations, and should strive to maintain 'the process of life' and not 'the process of dying'. At a meeting in Amman, Jordan in 1986, the Islamic Fiqh Academy (IFA, the international body of Islamic scholars and jurists) and the Organization of the Islamic Conference (OIC) reached a decision that death is declared when the 'heart or breath', or 'mental function', has stopped and is irreversible, essentially accepting neurological criteria for death. Hence the Kuwait and IFA-OIC decisions provide guidance that, although life cannot be discontinued if there is a possibility of recovery, withdrawing futile treatment (including ventilation) is permissible when death is imminent or is diagnosed by brain death criteria. However, these decisions are non-binding guidelines and, though accepted by the majority of Muslim doctors and scholars, consensus is not unanimous.

Buddhism[8]

There are over 500 million people in the world (or 7% of the world population) who are Buddhists. Buddhism is based on the teachings of Siddhartha Gautama, the Buddha, an Indian prince in the 6th century BCE. It became popular and spread from India to China, Japan, Tibet, Thailand, Sri Lanka and other Asian countries. Variances in schools and subschools developed, practised together with cultural customs, local deities, indigenous traditions (such as *feng shui* in China and *shinto* in Japan) and philosophical traditions, particularly Confucianism and Taoism in China. In Chinese traditions, filial piety and worship of ancestors are important. Complex rituals are believed to help the passage of the deceased from death to the status of ancestor and thus ensure harmony. Shinto traditions revere life, purity and nature; concepts like brain death are controversial, being difficult to reconcile as 'natural' proceedings. Tibetan Buddhism is blended with shamanic beliefs and practices as reflected in the book, *The Tibetan Book of the Dead*, to be read at the bedside of the dying. Western types of Buddhism with converted followers tend to focus on meditation more than ritual.

There is no 'one' Buddhist religion. The two main schools, Theravada and Mahayana, agree on the core teachings of the Buddha, but with some different expressions. Theravada Buddhism is associated with South East Asia and is perhaps closer to the original Indian form of Buddhism. Mahayana Buddhism, associated with Tibet, China and Japan, took on more local customs. Buddhism believes that every individual experiences the continual cycle of rebirths – *samsara* – which is influenced by *karma*, the natural consequences of the person's actions in the previous life. The state of a person's mind at the time of death and the karmic credit they have earned in life will determine the type of rebirth they will experience. Believers focus on personal spiritual development, aiming to attain a state of perfect peace, a mental and physical state known as *Nirvana* or Enlightenment (especially at the point of death), which will finally free them from the cycle of rebirths. The main sources of ethical guidance are the Three Jewels of Buddhism: the Buddha, the Dhamma (the Buddha's teaching) and the Sangha (the community of followers – monks and laity). Authoritarian statements are few, as Buddhism emphasises the necessity of discovering one's own path in life.

Three criteria in Buddhism distinguish a living body from a dead body: vitality, heat and consciousness. Today, vitality might resemble the body's metabolic processes and heat the energy generated by these processes – a set of metaphysical criteria which cannot be used in medicine to declare death. Buddhist acceptance of brain death is debatable, but some recognise this declaration of death for the purposes of organ donation because the latter is a generous, compassionate act to benefit others. In Buddhism, death and preparation for death are important. The state of the patient's mind (conscious, calm, meditative and peaceful) are crucial to dying in fulfilment; sedation and pain relief medications may need careful consideration. Withdrawing ventilation and life support treatment (including tube feeding) when death is imminent are accepted. Buddhism respects the dying process, and withdrawing futile treatment is to return the patient to a natural process of dying. Some Buddhists believe that the body should be left undisturbed and with minimal direct physical contact for a number of hours after death. This is, of course, almost always impractical in a busy, modern, acute hospital ward.

Hinduism[9]

There are about 1.15 billion people in the world who are Hindus, or 15% of the world population. Hinduism, the oldest known religion – since 1900–1400 BCE – and the majority religion in India and Nepal, is a fusion of various Indian cultures and traditions with no single founder or source. Hindus believe in one God, Brahman, manifested in many forms for believers to choose to worship. Scriptures, tradition, gurus and one's station in life provide guidance on moral behaviour. Like Buddhism, the Hindu religion believes in *karma* and rebirths. A good life with good deeds and devotion to God, ending in a good death, will generate good *karma* that will lead to a good rebirth, and a better status, spiritually and in life. Hindus, also like Buddhists, aim for attainment of Enlightenment, or *moksha,* to end the cycle of rebirths.

The vast majority of Hindus live in India. Subsequently, Indian laws and customs influence Hindu ethical considerations in end-of-life care. Most Indians die at home, many being discharged from hospital as death nears – one reason for the scarcity of discussions on religious aspects of care of the dying. In Hinduism, suicide and euthanasia are morally wrong. Indian law accepts brain death criteria, and there are references in Hindu scriptures that support the concept of organ donation. However, many Hindus are uncomfortable with the concept of brain death. Nonetheless, Hinduism can accept withdrawing or withholding futile treatment despite an absence of guidelines in Indian laws. Futile treatment, such as continuing ventilation, can be viewed as interfering with the timing of natural death, thus leading to an eventual bad death, with consequences of bad *karma* for the patient and bad luck for the family. Those Hindus, whether born or converted, who live outside India may have different interpretations of Hinduism on issues relating to end-of-life care.

*

'Very heavy, very interesting, Tom', Mike said, cocking his head, eyebrows raised. I wasn't sure if he meant it; he hadn't looked too interested. 'But what happens in reality … in practice really, in the hospital? How do you handle a hard-core fundamentalist family member?'

'In reality, families overall appreciate the care given to their loved ones, and uncommonly raise problems because of their religious convictions. Good communication is key. If need be, we involve social workers and experts, either hospital volunteers or the family's minister, priest or clergy. Respect for their beliefs is central', I said. 'We try to follow the triple 'C' doctrine … the Church of Compassion and Common sense.'

'And thank God for that!'

*

Reflections

- Healthcare staff should have some understanding of the major religions in their population area, and must respect faiths and beliefs of others.
- Healthcare staff should understand preferences in medical care that are influenced by the patient's religion.
- In general, the major religions do not hinder modern medical practices in recognising brain death, withdrawing futile treatment, and organ donation.
- Good communication with families is a key approach.

References

1. Puchalski M, O'Donnell E. Religious and spiritual beliefs in end of life care: how major religions view death and dying. *Tech Reg Anesth Pain Manag* 2005;9(3):114–21.
2. *Views on end-of-life medical treatments. religion and public life.* Washington, DC: Pew Research Centre; 2013.

3. Setta SM, Shemie SD. An explanation and analysis of how world religions formulate their ethical decisions on withdrawing treatment and determining death. *Philos Ethics Humanit Med* 2015;10:6.
4. Romaina M, Sprung CL. Approaches to patients and families with strong religious beliefs regarding end-of-life care. *Curr Opin Crit Care* 2014;20:668–72.
5. Linzer RD. Treatment of terminally ill patients according to Jewish law. *Virtual Mentor* 2013;13(12):1081–7.
6. Andruchow B. *Medical bioethics: an Orthodox Christian perspective for Orthodox Christians. Family Life*, vol. III. Syosset, NY: Orthodox Church in America; 2010.
7. Bloomer MJ, Al-Mutair A. Ensuring cultural sensitivity for Muslim patients in the Australian ICU: considerations for care. *Aust Crit Care* 2013;26(4):193–6.
8. McCormick AJ. Buddhist ethics and end-of-life care decisions. *J Soc Work End Life Palliat Care* 2013;9(2–3):209–25.
9. Sharma H, Jagdish V, Anusha P, Bharti S. End-of-life care: Indian perspective. *Indian J Psychiatry* 2013;55(Suppl. 2):S293–8.

13

Cultures and ethnicities

Different from us

One of the great things about Sydney is that it has a great acceptance of everyone and everything. It's an incredibly tolerant city, a city with a huge multicultural basis.

Baz Luhrmann (1962–), Australian film director,
screenwriter and producer

*

With religion, the culture and ethnicity of patients and their families can influence their preferences in end-of-life care. The values of many ethnic and culturally diverse groups may at times be in conflict with our society's core values, such as patient autonomy. Such conflicting values can lead to miscommunication, fragmented, inadequate or inappropriate care and a poor death for the patient. Better awareness of cultures and ethnicities – '*cultural competency*' – is an accepted need for healthcare staff in delivering end-of-life care.

*

She stood beaming with three patients in hospital pyjamas at the front entrance to the hospital: a young Aboriginal man, a young woman from Somali and, in front of them, an elderly Chinese woman in a wheelchair. This was the photo of Ms Anne Di Costo, the hospital's public relations director, on the front page of the monthly hospital newsletter. The article was titled 'Multicultural Australia' and it described Ms Di Costo's account of how the hospital had achieved 'cultural competence' to become 'ethnic friendly'. But it was not always so, as reflected by the story that Dr Milton Frank, our senior consultant, had told me.

*

The fall of Saigon – the capital of South Vietnam, now called Ho Chi Minh City – to communist North Vietnam in April 1975 ended the Vietnam War. It also triggered a new worldwide phenomenon: that of boat people, a mass exodus of refugees fleeing their homeland (and for their lives) by sea in small boats for safer shores. Most of us welcomed the first boats that landed in Australia. After all, these were our compatriots in the fight against the commies. This notion was supported and promoted by the media, with photos of welcoming officials, one showing an immigration officer with his arms laden with teddy bears for the kids. Then more and more boats arrived, and the tide of media and public opinion turned. Who were these illegal immigrants, economic refugees, queue-jumpers, Asians, coming unscreened by boat? We will decide who comes to our country.

Around this time, we admitted a young 'boat woman' with the common surname Nguyen. We called her 'June', the month of her arrival, because we could not pronounce her given names. June had survived her hazardous journey, but when she should have been safe, had contracted pneumonia at the refugee camp. A camp officer brought her husband to see her twice a week. Mr Nguyen was a young man who had been a soldier in the South Vietnamese army. He spoke little English and we had no hospital interpreters then. Dressed in poor-fitting donated clothes, and with matted, greasy hair, he looked unkempt. He kept bowing to all staff members without saying a word, all the time with an impassive face, the archetypal 'inscrutable oriental', a common derogatory term used by Australians for Asians. June's condition deteriorated. Her pneumonia was viral in origin, making antibiotics ineffective. Her oxygenation continued to worsen despite ventilation and she soon developed multiorgan failure. Three weeks after her admission, we managed to convey to her husband and camp authorities that her death was imminent. A few hours before she died, Mr Nguyen walked in with a 10-month-old baby that we knew nothing about. It was their boy who had miraculously survived the rickety boat journey when others had died.

When June died, Nguyen's impassive face cracked. He sat beside her bed, with his torso slumped on top of her, cradling the baby in one arm and hugging his dead wife in the other. Now momentarily free of cultural inhibitions, he sobbed uncontrollably. The baby kicked his legs and broke into a smile. Then, everyone started crying, without exception, sharing his loss. We had not known how to manage him, being always polite, helpful and coolly professional towards him, but nothing more. Our cultural incompetence had blinded us, and we could not see past our society's prejudices. They were just like us and we felt that we had let them down.

*

The White Australia Policy that barred people of non-European descent from immigrating to Australia was introduced soon after

1901, when Australia became a federation. After World War II it was gradually dismantled and in 1973–75 the Whitlam Government made racial discrimination unlawful in selecting immigrants. Up to the 1970s, the Australian population was overwhelmingly Caucasian, and not the multiracial and multicultural society it is today. Cultural incompetence was excusable then, but not now, especially in our conduct towards dying patients and their families who are not Caucasians or Western-cultured Australians.

Culture and ethnicity are interrelated. Culture is the sum of socially transmitted beliefs, behaviour patterns, arts, institutions and products of labour and thought that reflect a particular community, population, class or period. Ethnicity relates to classifying mankind into groups based on racial, linguistic, religious and other common characteristics. Although ethnicity and race share an ideology of common ancestry, they differ in that race is primarily unitary. You can have only one race (even if it is mixed), regardless of location, but you can claim multiple ethnic affiliations. For example, Anne Di Costo, who was born and raised in Queensland, has an Italian father and extended family, and a mother from Northern Ireland. She is culturally Australian, with Italian and Irish ethnicities, and is a Caucasian by race. Nationality is the term generally accepted as the country of citizenship or permanent residence, and she can claim triple nationalities: Australian, Italian and British. The terms 'culture', 'ethnicity' and 'race' are not directly interchangeable, but the term 'cultural competence' is often used to encompass these issues.

Culture and ethnicity in healthcare define how the patient and family receive information, perceive proposed treatment and conduct communication, and what expectations they may harbour.[1] Cultural diversity is moderated by better education, higher social economic status and acculturation, but may be more pronounced by gender and paternalism issues. Although healthcare staff cannot be expected to know the intricacies of how different cultures express behaviour in the face of death, understanding some basics will help families to cope with dying in a respectful manner. Culture subsumes some beliefs from religion and, in general, there are common points of cultural diversity with Western medicine. These issues can be viewed under the areas of medical care, communication and family (*see Box 1*).

| 1. Cultural Diversity in Healthcare ||
Culture of Western medicine	Other cultures
• Autonomy, individualism	• Collectivism
• Full disclosure	• Withholding bad news
• Patient is sole decision maker	• Family role in decision making
• Control in decision making	• Reluctance in decision making
• Direct communication	• Circuitous communication
• Avoiding futile treatment	• Advocacy in greater intervention
• Scientific/technological approach to EoL	• Spiritual/faith-based approach to EoL
• Avoidance of pain	• Cultural significance of pain
• Death is EoL	• Views on afterlife

EoL, end of life.

Autonomy

Many cultures do not value autonomy over beneficence, seeing patient welfare as being more important than empowerment. Collective decision making is more the norm in many cultures than the patient's individual right. Some cultures, such as in South East Asia, respect learned authority and attribute a high degree of deference to doctors. Patients and families concede end-of life decisions to the doctor – who is seen as an expert – tending not to ask questions or articulate disagreements. Mr Nguyen expressed this behaviour. Nonetheless, there may be reluctance for some medical interventions in end-of-life-care, with prefer-ence sometimes for non-Western medicine techniques such as herbal remedies. Some people from countries with authoritarian regimes may mistrust doctors and the health system altogether. Culture can also affect a person's response to pain, in the meaning and expression of pain. Pain may be welcomed as a positive symptom, or as a test of one's faith through suffering, or even as a punishment; asking for pain medication may be considered a sign of weakness or as going against nature. Indeed, the patient and family may feel shame and guilt about the illness. The acceptance of advance care directives or living wills varies among cultures.

Family

Family and extended family ties are extremely important in many cultures. Decisions will often be family orientated, to remove that burden from the patient. In some Asian and Eastern European cultures, paternalism, or decision making by the head of family, is the norm; with many Indians, the eldest son holds pole position in the family if the father is the patient. Family-based medical decisions are a function of filial piety among Asian cultures, particularly the Chinese and followers of Confucianism. This reverence for parents and elders who are sick drives beneficence. To do good to benefit the elder patient, families may insist that all medical interventions be delivered, even in end-of-life care.

Filial piety may also be a factor for Asians to avoid telling the truth about the illness and prognosis to the patient. Western medicine values autonomy, the patient's right to be informed of the illness and treatment options, and to choose or refuse medical care. Many cultures, however, often conceal bad news from the patient out of respect, and to protect against anxiety and depression that may eliminate hope. Indeed, many patients, families and even doctors in south-eastern Europe, much of Asia, Central and South America and the Middle East feel withholding medical information is a more humane approach.

Deeply religious groups, such as Catholic Filipinos, believe that death is a fate in the hands of God and bad news can be self-fulfilling. Western medicine, in general, discounts the importance of religion and spirituality but some cultures, irrespective of faith, believe that God, and not doctors, has the ultimate say in life and death, and that suffering may be redemptive and should be endured.

To lay people, medical terminology is a foreign language. Moreover, to families who do not speak English (or the host language) – like Mr Nguyen – language is a massive barrier in communication. Also, in communicating with Asians, *face* or public dignity is important. To make a family member *lose face,* such as by showing up the eldest son's ignorance of an issue in front of the family, is to cause him humiliation and loss of prestige. On the family side, a member may not tell the full truth, for fear of losing face by giving wrong or indelicate information. Although more of a religious request than one of cultural practice when death is near, some families may ask for a religious representative to be present at the bedside to perform a ritual. How the body is handled, washed or viewed after death may be important.

Indigenous cultures

The culture of indigenous people is influenced by the dominant society. One example is Australia's indigenous people, Australian Aborigines and Torres Strait Islanders,[2] who make up 2.5% of the population. The latter – from the Torres Strait Islands, which separate north Australia from New Guinea – are genetically Melanesian (the same as Papua New Guineans), and racially and culturally distinct from Australian Aborigines. Both share an identity: that of colonisation by Britain and Christian missionaries, with dispossession, oppression and suppression of their traditional cultures. Their remaining practices, albeit influenced by Christianity with regard to Torres Strait Islanders, differ from those of Australia's Western society.

Australia's indigenous people have a strong spiritual connection with land and water, and storytelling in families is an important traditional way to maintain these connections. Spiritual beliefs also often explain causes of poor health, with different interpretations about diagnoses. A hospital may be seen more as a place to die than a place to be healed. Communication can be difficult for staff. English is not always a spoken language, and both indigenous cultures show a reluctance to accept bad news or prognoses. In Aboriginal culture, on particular topics, it is preferable for men to speak to men – 'men's business' – and for women to speak to women – 'women's business'. Personal questions can raise suspicion. An Aboriginal or Torres Strait Islander patient may not express their level of pain experienced because of embarrassment. Families and elders are important in both cultures. In Aboriginal culture, the extended family will need to be informed and consulted for decision making by the community. When death occurs, there is a nominated person to contact – not necessarily the next-of-kin – who will inform the family when the patient dies. It is sometimes inappropriate for a staff member to do this, especially a non-Aboriginal person. This spiritual connection with the land and some other cultural aspects, such as the importance of family, elders and traditions, are also seen in indigenous groups of other countries, such as North American Indians and New Zealand Māoris.[1]

After death

Following death, some cultures have important beliefs and rituals to uphold. In Jewish mourning tradition, the body is not viewed and there are no flowers near the deceased. Many cultures believe that after death the spirit is released from the body to continue to the next stage of the afterlife journey. Improper observations of traditional rituals will disable this journey, consequently causing disruption to the family. Australian Aboriginals forbid taking images of and writing or speaking the name of the deceased, to prevent interference with the journey. Relatives of the deceased expect staff to avoid eye contact with them following the patient's death as a mark of respect. An expectation for immediate and extended family members to gather at the bedside is common, as is dying at home or returning to the homeland after death. Many cultures believe in proper funeral rituals to free the spirit.

Communication

The basics of effective communication (Chapter 7 Communication) and attention to the issues in Box 1 are important when communicating with culturally diverse patients or their families. If available and necessary, the help of interpreters and cultural experts should be arranged early. Staff should convey empathy and show interest in the family's cultural heritage for family members to feel more comfortable. Evaluating the family's socio-economic background will help in understanding their concerns and to gain an insight into their values, spirituality, relationship dynamics and acculturation. Doctors should explain why ethical and professional obligations are necessary in medical care, such as autonomy and informed consent, and the reasons why certain requests cannot be implemented, such as continuing treatment after brain death has been confirmed. In return, by asking questions of the family (*see Box 2*), their preferences will be known. Family members may convey their feelings by non-verbal clues, such as facial expressions and voice tone, without making explicit statements.

Staff must always avoid stereotyping a group or an individual. A patient or family may not necessarily follow the traditions known for that cultural group; for example, an 'inscrutable oriental' may turn out to be a local-born, educated professional. Stereotyping patients is simply medical race profiling. Greeting a family with one or two words in their language that one knows, to make

2. Patient-centred Questions Concerning Patient and Family

Religion
What religion? How religious?

Medical information and decision making
With patient only? With patient and family? With family only?
Who to contact? Who is next of kin?
How much to know? Non-disclosure (not all truth)? Views on futile
   treatment?

Presence of others in discussions
Interpreters? Priests, ministers, etc.? Family members, friends?

Specific issues
What are important? What are difficult to discuss?

Advance directive
Is there one? What are specified?

Requests
Pain management? Special requests? More questions?

By eliciting and following cultural preferences that relate to seriously ill
patients, staff can provide culturally-sensitive end-of-life care.

them feel comfortable (and to show off) can be regarded as
gratuitous and patronising, likely to offend an educated family.
Similarly, speaking English slowly to make them understand better
is demeaning theatre. At all times, staff should understand and
respect the patient and family and their wishes. Cultural competence will help guide the dying patient die a good death.

I wonder what became of Mr Nguyen and his baby son?

*

Reflections

- Australia is a multicultural and multiracial society. Patients making
  their end-of-life journey and their families reflect this.
- Healthcare staff should have an understanding of the values of
  the major cultural and ethnic groups in their community.
- Race stereotyping and profiling, even with good intentions, is
  gratuitous, patronising and demeaning.
- A rule of thumb for all health professionals is: respect each
  other's values.

References

1. Coolen PR. *Cultural relevance in end-of-life care*. 1 May 2012. https://ethnomed.org.
2. Queensland Health. *Sad news, sorry business: guidelines for caring for Aboriginal and Torres Strait Islander people through death and dying*. Brisbane, QLD: Queensland Health; 2015. www.health.qld.gov.au/.../151736/sorry_business.pdf.

References

PART VI

Health Services

14

The healthcare system

Navigating the healthcare maze

The current health care system is neither healthy, caring, nor a system.

Walther Cronkite (1916–2009), American journalist and TV commentator, on the US health system

Hospitals are highly complex, small societies, unknowable by any one individual … Most families struggle to understand the teams, sites, sounds, language, and personnel inside what they see as a strange and sometimes terrifying place … Most of them have only vague knowledge, if any, of human physiology and disease, medical procedures, or those organizational features of the hospital that determine what happens to patients.

Sharon Kaufman (1948–), American medical anthropologist, in her book '*… And a time to die*' (2005)[1]

*

When patients are admitted into hospital, they and their families enter an alien environment that is disconnected from

175

their everyday lives. They meet a phalanx of doctors and nurses. They learn the name of their consultant specialist, but are confused by the organisation hierarchy, the lines of authority, the pecking order of doctors and nurses, and the roles of people in uniforms with clipboards. There are hospital routines that they must follow, with many procedures determined by patterns of hospital practice, a complicated system of rules known only to hospital staff. The route to recovery or death is influenced by the hospital culture, standards of care, health costs, fees and the hospital system, which is part of the healthcare system. In that journey, they encounter referrals to other specialists, transfers to different wards, investigations, treatment by different doctors and a myriad of bills from doctors that they do not know and for services about which they have no clue. Patients and families feel helpless, frustrated and guilty because of their overall lack of knowledge, adding to the stress that serious illness brings. They have questions regarding the illness, such as treatment choices and prognostic outcomes, but they also have questions regarding the healthcare system, such as, 'Who is the most experienced doctor for this condition? Can we choose this doctor? Which hospital has the best outcomes for this condition, and can we be transferred to this hospital? How do we get a second opinion? What are the costs of treatment? Who pays, and if we do, what are the fees?'

Knowing more about how your healthcare system will help you and your family navigate this maze when confronted by serious illness or when receiving end-of-life care.

*

Healthcare system

A healthcare system is the organisation of resources, institutions and health professionals to deliver health services to the population with three goals: to keep citizens healthy, to treat the sick and to protect them from extravagant health costs. Only developed countries have healthcare systems. Many countries are too poor or disordered to provide proper healthcare to the masses. Then only the rich have access to medical care.

A healthcare system has primary healthcare and secondary healthcare divisions. Primary healthcare describes 'family doctor' or general practitioner (GP) services delivered to individuals, but the division also includes 'public health' or population-level services. Secondary healthcare describes services delivered by medical specialists and other health professionals who do not have first contact with patients, with the initial referral made by the GP. Tertiary healthcare is a term sometimes used to describe advanced medical investigative and treatment services in tertiary teaching hospitals (sometimes called principal referral hospitals). For example, such hospitals deliver care in critical illness, major trauma, neurosurgery and cardiothoracic surgery.

Each country has its own system, but there are four basic models.[2]

1. *The National Health or Beveridge Model* is named after Lord Beveridge, who designed the UK's National Health Service (NHS). Healthcare is financed by the Government through taxes, and provided free in state-owned hospitals and clinics by salaried staff. No one is denied healthcare or receives a bill. Private medicine exists outside the NHS in doctors providing healthcare to fee-paying patients in private hospitals. The UK, Italy, Spain, Norway, Denmark, Finland, Sweden and New Zealand operate this system.

2. *The Bismarck Model*, named after the 19th-century Prussian Chancellor, uses an insurance system run by not-for-profit funds, paid for by joint contributions from employees and employers. Private doctors and hospitals generally provide the healthcare. Germany, France, Belgium, the Netherlands, Japan and Switzerland primarily use this system.

3. *The National Health Insurance Model* uses elements of the previous two systems. A taxpayer-funded, government-run insurance fund pays for healthcare services to private sector providers. Apart from simpler administration, the single fund has the economic power to negotiate lower costs, e.g. from pharmaceutical companies. This system is used by Canada, Taiwan and South Korea.

4. *The Private Insurance Model* uses insurance funds to pay for private healthcare. Private insurance is obtained through one's employer or through a private insurance company. Those with no insurance or government assistance are not covered for healthcare. This is an expensive out-of-pocket model, and is the major system in the US with its many systems for separate classes of people.

*

'Did you read Joan's article?', my wife Di asked. She was referring to the latest issue of '*Community news*', our suburban newspaper. We had met the journalist Joan Blade at a dinner at my neighbours' house. She wrote for the paper on health matters, and was a perennial fierce critic of the health system, particularly of doctors. The article reported on a number of recent mishaps – none major – at our city hospitals. She concluded with the advice to readers to 'choose your doctor and choose your hospital'.

*

Australian healthcare system[3]

Other countries have systems that utilise elements of government and private funding to offer public and private healthcare. Australia has such a mixed system, made complex by multiple providers and a variety of regulatory, multi-layered responsibilities of different jurisdictions (states and territories). Medicare, the national health insurance scheme, is funded through taxation to provide free or subsidised access to medical, diagnostic and allied health services. Patients pay for subsidised medicines dispensed by private community pharmacists under the government-funded Pharmaceutical Benefits Scheme.

Public hospital treatment is free, including medications, but patients with non-urgent conditions are likely to wait long periods for treatment. These cases are referred by GPs to outpatient clinics, and elective surgery and procedures are scheduled from the clinics' waiting lists. Patients with acute conditions, injuries or cancer are admitted through the emergency department and attended to without delay. Tertiary teaching (public) hospitals provide advanced services that private hospitals may not. Public hospitals employ salaried staff, and consultant specialists may be full time or part time. The latter also practise in outside private clinics and hospitals.

*

The phone call was from Joe Fitzgerald, one of the members in my cycling peloton. 'Tom? Joe here. Need help please. Dad is booked to have Whipple's surgery at St Mary's private hospital next month, by a surgeon Dr John Appleby. I'd rather you look after dad post surgery. He's got private insurance of course. Can you arrange this?'

I felt awkward. 'Sorry, Joe. No can do. I am not accredited at St Mary's. Your dad can be operated on at my hospital, but Appleby is not a consultant here and has no access. One of our surgeons can operate on him, if he comes in as a private patient, but he would have to join a waiting list. Also, ethically and professionally, I can't take over your dad's care from Appleby who, by the way, is a good surgeon', I said. This was a request that I infrequently receive from friends. A patient with private health insurance may choose to be treated as a private patient when admitted into a public hospital. This enables a choice of doctors (but only from those on the hospital staff) and better 'hotel' benefits. However, no private patient can be admitted directly from home to bypass waiting lists, unless the illness is urgent.

*

Private hospitals cater to patients who want a choice of doctor and ward accommodation. The chosen doctor can only treat patients in the private hospital that accredits him or her to practise. Thus a private patient's choice of doctor may not align with the choice of hospital. Medicare pays a proportion of the private doctors' fees, and private health insurance covers most of the private hospital fees. Insured consumers can avoid long queues of public hospitals by being treated in private facilities. Private health insurance also provides cover for many out-of-hospital services not covered by Medicare, such as dentistry.

The states and territories are responsible for managing public hospitals (which are jointly funded with the Commonwealth), public health services and community health facilities. Public hospitals have organised clinical departments according to medical specialties. Each department's medical pecking order is: a head of department, consultant specialists, registrars who are training to be specialists, resident medical officers, who are waiting to be registrars, and interns, first-year medical graduates, who are the bottom of the food chain. Patients are admitted under the consultant team on duty that day. Public patients may not choose their doctor, and may not request transfer to another hospital unless the move is to the private sector or to a public special care facility. Consultants may seek advice from colleagues of other specialty departments on managing conditions outside their expertise. Any request for a second opinion from a patient or family is directed to the consultant in charge, who then arranges a colleague to review the case. Public patients will not receive any invoice for their hospital stay. Those who choose to be admitted as private patients will be billed for medical and bed fees. These are reimbursed in part by Medicare and the private health insurance fund respectively.

Comparisons of healthcare systems[4,5]

Studies on comparisons and ranking of healthcare systems among various developed countries have been published. A multitude of indicators have been used as datasets, including health funding, number of doctors and healthcare professionals, life expectancy, infant mortality rate, GDP per capita, healthcare expenditure as percentage of GDP, access, responsiveness, patient-centred care, safety, equity, outcomes and sustainability (cost to consumer and government). Conclusions can be considered of debatable usefulness, but Australia's system can be considered favourable.

*

Reflections

- Australia's healthcare system is a mixed bag of public and private medicine, managed under the regulations of many jurisdictions.
- Medicare (the government's tax-funded universal insurance fund) and private health insurance funds reimburse most of private doctors' fees and private hospital costs respectively.
- Healthcare in a public hospital is free but patients cannot choose their public hospital or doctor, and the waiting list for non-urgent care may be long.
- Patients and families should familiarise themselves with the workings of their local public and private hospitals and their medical teams to receive optimal care without ending in penury. Start with your GP.

References

1. Kaufman SR. ... *And a time to die. How American hospitals shape the end of life*. New York: Simon & Shuster; 2005.
2. Wallace LS. A view of health care around the world. *Ann Fam Med* 2013;11(1):84.
3. Australian Institute of Health and Welfare. *Australia's health 2014*. Australia's health series no. 14. Canberra: AIHW; 2014.
4. Braithwaite J, Hibbert P, Blakely B, Plumb J, Hannaford N, Long JC, et al. Health system frameworks and performance indicators in eight countries: a comparative international analysis. *SAGE Open Med* 2017;5:2050312116686516.
5. Papanicolas I, Smith PC, editors. *Health system performance analysis – an agenda for policy, information and research*. Maidenhead, Berks, UK: Open University Press / McGraw-Hill Education; 2013.

15

The intensive care unit

Intensive, expensive care

A good intensive care specialist must have:
- *The keen observation of a paediatrician (ventilated ICU patients cannot talk).*
- *The patience of an obstetrician (watchful waiting is a part of beneficial therapy).*
- *The thoughtfulness of a physician (multiple complex problems need sorting).*
- *The rapid reflexes of an anaesthesiologist (quick thinking and action as needed).*
- *The aggressiveness of a surgeon (definitive invasive intervention when needed).*
- *The communication skills of a psychiatrist (families and friends need counselling).*[1]

Dr A.K. Khanna and Dr L.J. Kaplan, American Society of Critical Care Medicine (2015)

*

The intensive care unit (ICU) is also known as the intensive therapy unit or critical care unit. It is a specially designed and staffed ward that treats patients with severe and life-threatening illnesses and injuries. These patients receive constant monitoring and physiological support using specialised equipment and medications, under the charge of intensive care specialists called intensivists and dedicated ICU nurses. It is commonly the 'twilight zone' setting.

*

Dr Rachel Lim waited. The ICU doors burst open and the bed trolley surged through, pushed by the burly orderly and flanked on the left by the emergency department nurse, her right hand on the bed rail. Her other hand clutched the admission notes against her chest. A skinny man with black curly hair followed – the emergency department intern – giving off a worldly and disinterested air in his floral shirt and jeans. The obese, middle-aged patient in the trolley sat bolt upright, with laboured, noisy breathing and bulging neck muscles. His blue shirt was bathed with sweat, with front buttons undone. An oxygen mask sat on his bloated, sickly, blue-grey face.

Rachel Lim watched the entourage trundle hurriedly past patients in the bed bays. Startled relatives looked up with some unease, more so when the obese man became agitated. Too breathless to shout, he shook his head side to side, thrashed his legs and repeatedly tried to rip off his oxygen mask. The intern kept restraining him without success.

The trolley stopped at bay 5, near the end of the ward where Rachel Lim was waiting with three ICU nurses – Jane, Mary and Rosemary Smith, the charge nurse. The intern suddenly shouted with a nervous shrill to nobody in particular, 'Jim Rastor 55, respiratory failure!' Everyone ignored him as they helped the orderly heave the struggling, obese man from the trolley across to the ICU bed, a laudable feat. Rosemary drew the bed curtains. Mary gently shepherded the intern out of the way. Rachel positioned herself behind the man.

'Jim, I'm Dr Lim', she said. 'You're in ICU now. I need to put you on our breathing machine, but first I need to put you to sleep. Don't worry, you'll be OK.' There was no time for fine bedside manners. The man was in no state to disapprove. Rachel noticed the sweat-matted, white hair at the back of the head and the nicotine-stained fingers. She quickly replaced the oxygen mask with the resuscitator bag mask to deliver 100% oxygen. Jane fiddled with the ventilator dials, setting volume, frequency and oxygen concentration. Mary applied the blood pressure cuff on Jim's left arm, and stuck ECG electrodes on his hairy chest. She clipped the pulse oximeter stall on his right index finger. The big colour monitor sprang to life. A green ECG line skipped with heartbeats, showing a rapid rate of 180 per minute. A blue '*200/110 mmHg*' told of a high blood pressure. The pulse oximeter bleeped and blinked brightly in red – '*saturation 85%*' – a dangerously low blood oxygen level. Rosemary had by now moved the intravenous (IV) fluid bags from the trolley to the ICU bed pole. She untangled the IV lines to determine which venous access to inject the drugs that were lined up on a tray.

Jim's phlegm-congested coughing jolted Rachel. 'Ready?', she asked. The nurses nodded. 'Midazolam 15 milligrams over 20 seconds', she ordered and Rosemary injected the sleep-inducing drug into the right arm IV. Jim collapsed back on to the sweat-drenched bed, no longer struggling. Rachel immediately lowered the backrest to lay him flat. 'Scoline 100 milligrams', she requested. Susan injected the muscle relaxant and quickly applied cricoid pressure. This firm pressure on Jim's Adam's apple with thumb and index finger occludes stomach contents from regurgitating into the trachea to soil the lungs. Rachel inserted the laryngoscope into Jim's mouth. The foetid odour momentarily gagged her. She suctioned the copious secretions in the oral cavity while holding her breath. When she visualised the vocal cords, she passed the endotracheal tube into the trachea. Susan inflated the cuff of the endotracheal tube to seal off the trachea, and connected it to the ventilator before deftly securing it with tapes.

Jim's airway was now safeguarded and the ventilator was delivering adequate breaths to his wrecked, congested lungs. It was a brief undertaking, over in minutes and carried out with professional skill. I had stood by and my assistance was not needed. The pulse oximeter readings began to rise slowly … 86% … 88% … 90%, and the improving oxygenation was reflected in Jim's skin colour. The intern watched dourly in awe. Everyone began to feel good. Tension palpably melted.

'Thanks guys, well done', Rachel said, pleased and relieved. 'I'll insert an arterial line and CVP when you're ready. Standard blood tests please, and micro specimens. Might as well book the chest CT as well as chest X-ray.' She checked the ventilator settings, and then listened to Jim's chest. His ventilated breaths sounded like a sonorous brass band, completely out of tune. 'Let's get the physios. I'll write the forms and antibiotics later.' The emergency department nurse handed over details to Jane, and Mary began to clean up.

Rachel turned to the intern and said, 'You did well, sitting Mr Rastor upright ... better gas exchange in patients with respiratory failure.' He hunched his shoulders and glowered sullenly, suspicious of the compliment. Rachel had given a tutorial the previous week to the hospital interns on 'oxygen therapy'. *It benefited this intern obviously. Why do they dress like 19th-century mental asylum escapees?*

*

Intensive care units

Jim Rastor was one of 150,000 Australians who receive hospital ICU care each year. If he were to eventually die from his respiratory failure, he would be among 12,000 Australians who die each year in the ICU, or 8.6% of all ICU admissions,[2] and a significant 13% of all hospital deaths. Astoundingly, almost a quarter of all deaths in the US occur in or after admission to an ICU.[3] Hence end-of-life care is an important component of ICU care. As most people in developed countries die in hospitals, the ICU is commonly the last stop in our travel through the twilight zone. How ICUs operate should thus be of interest to many of us.

Origins of ICUs

Several key people contributed to the development of ICUs and intensive care medicine. Florence Nightingale, serving in the Crimean War (1850–54), placed the frailest soldiers closest to her nursing station where she could provide better care. Following this concept, in the 1940s some US and European hospitals established a 'recovery' area next to the operating rooms to care for surgical patients in the immediate postoperative period. This gave impetus to a similar concept for the whole hospital: the ICU. The Danish polio epidemic of 1952 was a keystone event in founding ICUs.[4] Hundreds of victims were hospitalised, in respiratory failure and drowning in their secretions. The few inefficient 'iron lung' tank respirators available could not cope, and over 80% of patients died. A Copenhagen anaesthetist, Dr Björn Ibsen, engaged medical students to hand-ventilate victims in a special ward using rubber breathing bags, and he decreased mortality by half. Harry Weil in California, US, established a 'shock ward' during the early 1960s, considered a forerunner of ICUs. Peter Safar, an anaesthetist, established the concept of 'advanced support of life' in the 1950s and opened the first multidisciplinary ICU in the world in Baltimore, Maryland, US, in 1958. Similarly, advances in cardiac surgery in the 1960s also promoted special care in an ICU.

Over the following 30 years, ICUs became established world-wide and intensive care grew into the multidisciplinary specialty today, and the role of the specialist intensivist became recognised. In Australia and New Zealand, certification by the College of Anaesthetists (now taken over by the College of Intensive Care Medicine) is an example. Cardiac or coronary care units and paediatric ICUs likewise evolved with general ICUs. Many hospitals, particularly in the US, also developed subspecialty ICUs, such as the medical ICU, surgical ICU, cardiothoracic ICU and neurosurgical ICU, staffed primarily by their specialty doctors. Obviously, subspecialty ICUs require more beds and resources, but benefits in terms of patient outcome compared with care in general ICUs are debatable.

ICU casemix

Many articles and stories on end-of-life care concern the elderly and the chronically infirmed in nursing care, and geriatric and palliative care institutions. In contrast, ICU patients are younger, with trauma and injury victims making up a significant demographic group. The casemix is thus dissimilar to a palliative care ward, and these ICU deaths have a different dying trajectory to those of most hospital patients. For example, a common trajectory of death is long-term debility with periods of acute exacerbation of symptoms, ending with a short period of decline. This is seen in chronic illness such as chronic obstructive pulmonary disease. The trajectory of cancers is that of a long period of relative stability followed by a short one of physical decline. Degenerative diseases (e.g. Alzheimer's, multiple sclerosis) have a trajectory of increasing frailty and loss of function. In the ICU, dying starts at the final stages of disease, or follows acute severe injuries, and the death trajectory has a short timespan. Hence the ICU's end-of-life care has its own challenging nuances. Some patient choices for dying, such as to die at home or from assisted suicide, are unrealistic in the ICU, if not impractical or illegal. Undoubtedly, the advanced state-of-the-art medicine practised in the ICU have saved more lives, but at a higher cost of care in money and in escalating interventions, giving rise to more potential ethical dilemmas. The ICU today is a rich window through which to view end-of-life scenarios, miraculous survivals, emotions and the resiliency of the human spirit.

Standards for ICUs

Standards for ICUs have been promulgated,[5] such as clinical and staffing guidelines of the Australian Council on Healthcare Standards. The numbers of beds depend upon the functional level (see below), size of the hospital, its casemix and its catchment region, and may range from 6 to over 40. The complexity of equipment will also be appropriate to the role of the ICU.

Appropriate nurse staffing depends on how the ICU functions. Patients needing complex management require higher nurse:patient ratios. The nurses are certified in intensive care nursing. Intensivists provide the medical care to the patients, but, in smaller ICUs, anaesthetists or respiratory physicians may help in after-hours rosters. Other staff members, depending on the needs of the ICU, include secretaries, physiotherapists, radiographers, dietitians, technicians and social workers.

Levels of ICUs

There are three levels of a general ICU for adult patients, defined according to the type of facility, care given, clinical standards and staffing requirements.

A *level 3 ICU* is a 'full-bottle' centre of excellence, capable of providing complex, multisystem life support for an indefinite period. It is located in a tertiary hospital with extensive backup of 'super-specialised' clinical and laboratory services.

A *level 2 ICU* provides 'general' intensive care services; specialised and backup clinical and laboratory services are not extensive. Most consultants are qualified specialist intensivists. It is located in a metropolitan or regional general hospital.

A *level 1 ICU* provides basic multisystem life support (mechanical ventilation and simple invasive cardiovascular monitoring) for less than 24 hours. It is found in a regional small hospital, or a small metropolitan private hospital. Consultants are not necessarily specialist intensivists. A patient who requires continuing intensive care will be transferred to a level 2 or level 3 ICU.

Some tertiary hospitals also have a *high-dependency unit* (HDU), which is operationally under the ICU team. This is a special ward that provides intermediate care between ICU care and general ward care – that is, as a step-down ward for uncomplicated recovering ICU patients and a spillover ward when the ICU is full.

Patients in public hospital ICUs are admitted from the emergency department, the wards or the operating theatres, and never from home. Both public and private hospitals in Australia have ICUs. In general, private ICUs do not admit seriously ill or injured patients *de novo*, and certainly not public patients. Their admissions are mostly elective, following major surgery at their hospital, or from an emergency event within the hospital stay. Private hospital ICUs are mostly level 1 or HDUs.

*

Reflections

- The ICU cares for critically ill patients who may proceed to end of life.
- Skilled specialist doctors and nurses in the ICU provide appropriate, sensitive end-of-life care.
- ICU care is expensive care.
- Patients cannot choose admission into a public or private ICU.

References

1. Khanna AK, Kaplan LJ. *Society of Critical Care Medicine archives 2015, 2nd April.*
2. Centre for Outcome and Resource Evaluation Adult Patient Database (APD). *Activity report 2017–2018.* Melbourne, VIC: Australian and New Zealand Intensive Care Society; 2018.

3. Truog RD, Campbell ML, Curtis JR, Haas CE, Luce JM, Rubenfeld GD, et al. American Academy of Critical Care Medicine. Recommendations for end-of-life care in the intensive care unit: a consensus statement by the American College [corrected] of Critical Care Medicine. *Crit Care Med* 2008;36(3):953–63.
4. Lassen HCA. A preliminary report on the 1952 epidemic of poliomyelitis in Copenhagen with special reference to the treatment of acute respiratory insufficiency. *Lancet* 1953;1:37–41.
5. College of Intensive Care Medicine of Australia and New Zealand. *Minimum standards for intensive care units.* Melbourne, VIC: CICM; 2011.

16

Distributive justice
Sharing the shrinking cake

We are the richest country in the world. We spend more on healthcare than any other country. Yet we have the worst healthcare in the Western world. Come on. We can do better than this.

Michael Moore (1954–), American author and filmmaker, on US healthcare in his film 'Sicko' (2007)

*

Healthcare is expensive, with the highest costs consumed by the sickest, particularly during the last few months of life. *Distributive justice* in medicine is the fair and equitable distribution of scarce healthcare resources for all society's socioeconomic and population groups. How we travel in our life's last journey may depend on how the health-funding cake is divided where we live. So, to follow distributive justice, how should that cake be cut?

*

'I know what you said about futility and withdrawing treatment. But even if she only had a one per cent chance of survival, the ICU doctors could have at least kept her going, just in case – you never know. You would though, wouldn't you Tom?', Mike my neighbour said of withdrawing treatment on his grandmother who had suffered a massive stroke. He turned away before I could answer, to reach over to the portable cooler for another can of beer. 'You know Nana came over here the day before her stroke, for Angus's fifth birthday?', he changed the subject, perhaps knowing what my answer would be. He snapped open his beer can tab, settled back in his chair and gulped down a mouthful before breaking into a satisfied smile. 'She brought a chocolate cake, big cake for the ten kids here. But some kids ended up with small pieces … crumbs really, because Jonno's fat kid ate most of it', he said, chuckling.

Just like hospital politics, I thought. 'Mike', I replied, 'The size of Nana's cake and Jonno junior's appetite largely determines how far to continue Nana's treatment.'

*

Healthcare costs

Healthcare costs are a substantial expenditure for any country. Australia's annual expenditure in 2017–18 was 10% GDP or A$7485 per capita.[1] Annual data (2017) for New Zealand were 9.2% GDP or US$3937 per capita,[2] and for UK 9.6% GDP or US$3859 per capita.[2] The big daddy of them all is the US,[2] with 17.1% GDP or US$10,246 per capita for 2017, a whopping US$3.3 trillion total, equalling the combined spending of the next 10 biggest spenders. Australia's performance in terms of health expenditure and life expectancy compares well with first-world countries.

Hospitals, especially public acute care hospitals, are the most expensive healthcare component, with salaries topping costs at 60%–80% of budgets. The average daily cost per bed in an Australian hospital ranges widely (*see Table*).[3] For comparisons of costs of stay, admissions are 'weighted'; the complexity of treatment required with factors such as age and location is also considered. Thus, the healthcare we receive depends on budgets plus factors such as geography, size of jurisdictions, volume and complexity of services, industrial rulings (salaries and work practices) and, of course, efficiency, where length-of-stay days for specific procedures can be compared.

Acute Hospital Admissions in Australia 2017–18

Jurisdiction	No. of hospitals	No. of admissions	No. of weighted admissions	Complexity factor#	Average cost (A$)	
					Per admission	Per weighted admission
NSW	95	1,635,575	1,818,488	1.11	5267	4737
VIC	79	1,675,397	1,572,290	0.94	4282	4563
QLD	196	1,400,536	1,342,059	0.96	4523	4720
SA	20	379,722	405,894	1.07	6032	5644
WA	33	531,540	532,146	1.00	5827	5821
TAS	23	121,513	135,195	1.11	5772	5188
NT	5	165,704	98,297	0.59	3697	6231
ACT	2	109,135	114,802	1.05	5319	5057
National	**453**	**6,019,172**	**6,019,172**	**1.00**	**4855**	**4855**

In acute hospitals, ICUs beds are the most expensive to operate, costing three to six times more than an acute general hospital bed. Australia, the UK, New Zealand and most of Europe allocate 2%–5% of their total hospital beds as ICU beds, but this ratio in US is higher, from 5% to 20%. Wealthy European countries like Germany and Belgium follow the high American bed numbers.

A 2013 study found an ICU in the US costs 20%–30% of the total expenditure of its hospital, and intensive care costs 20% of the national healthcare costs.[4] The cost of an occupied ICU bed per day ranges from US$2000 to over US$5000. Of course, costs depend on the complexities of patients treated, as reflected in the category of the ICU.[a] More specialised ICUs have more staff (e.g. two nurses per patient ratio), and they use more expensive equipment, drugs and tests on sicker patients. Also, some doctors in any field may practise defensive medicine, where multiple diagnostic tests or treatments are performed to guard against the possibility of malpractice litigation, even though such interventions may not be clinically warranted. Higher expenditures are seen in the first two days of hospital admission, especially in the elderly and for those admitted to ICU. With the increase in our ageing population, there may be more admissions into ICU of patients older than 80 years, with poorer outcomes and at higher costs.[5]

High costs in any acute hospital are amplified if misguidedly used on futile treatment. In assessments of 1136 patients in five American ICUs in 2013, doctors reported delivering futile treatment to 11% and 'probably futile' treatment to 8.6%. The patients in the former group who received futile care occupied 6.7% of the total patient bed-days at 3.5% of the cost of treating all patients,[4] a sum of US$2.6 million for 123 patients over 3 months. An earlier US landmark study of 9105 patients with life-threatening diagnoses reported a 6-month mortality rate of 47%; patients who died, died at great expense with poor cost-effective outcomes that were worse than other expensive treatments, such as cardiac surgery.[6] For most cases, the doctors were able to deduce futility of ongoing treatment, but nonetheless struggled to implement withdrawing life-sustaining treatment.

---

[a] ICUs are categorised into five types: neonatal, paediatric and three adults: level 3, level 2 and level 1. Level 3 ICUs are highly specialised, and located in big hospitals (Chapter 15 The intensive care unit).

Resource allocation

How then should valuable resources in healthcare, particularly acute care medicine, be allocated? The allocation of healthcare resources involves different levels of decision making ranging from *macroallocation* of Nana's health cake at national, regional and hospital levels, to *microallocation* at the individual patient and doctor level. A high degree of government regulation and participation in health is unavoidable, and probably desirable for altruistic reasons, but normal market dynamics are missing, perhaps rendering them more susceptible to waste and ineffectiveness. At all levels, it is necessary to allocate resources fairly and justly without inequalities: the concept of *distributive justice*. But what is 'fair' or 'just', or 'equal'? Aristotle is quoted as having said, *'Justice is equality, but only for equals; and justice is inequality, but only for those who are unequal,'* and *'The worst form of inequality is to try to make unequal things equal.'*[7] He reasoned that, in a society, everyone could not fundamentally be equal. Distributive justice is not dividing resources equally, but rather justly and fairly involving the principle of *equitable distribution*, which means 'fair' division (as may be used to divide property in a divorce) and not numerically 'equal' division. Goods or resources are proportionately distributed according to impartial criteria, so that just shares are given on the basis of what one deserves or needs. The problem with equitable distribution is determining what criteria are morally relevant to distinguish a share that is proportionate (and thus deserving) from that which is disproportionate (and thus excessive or deficient). For example, if the ICU receives two requests for admission to the last-available ICU bed, what criteria should you use to decide which patient gets admitted?

Distributive justice principles

Theories with applicable principles have been proposed for equitable distribution (distributive justice) of healthcare resources that will impact on both macroallocation by society and micro-allocation at the individual patient level. These are:

1. *Egalitarian or treating people equally theory.* The egalitarian *lottery principle* supports an equal claim to resources but is impractical in acute admissions and care. The *first-come,*

first-served principle is generally applicable to walk-in outpatient and GP consultations, but it ignores relevant differences between people, and in practice fails to treat people fairly; queue jumping is possible. Also, with limited resources, should we apply egalitarian considerations to provide equal healthcare *access* or to achieve equal *outcomes* from treatment? How do we apply rationing equally?

2. *Utilitarian or maximising benefits theory. Save the most lives,* the ultimate utilitarian principle, is not practical in the ICU. It ignores people-factors – for example, whether three 80-year-olds who might each live for 5–10 more years is more worthy than one 20-year-old who might live another 60–70 years if saved. The *prognosis or life-years principle* excludes people with poor prognoses, such as barring them from organ transplant waiting lists. However, is giving many prognostic life-years to a few better than giving a few life-years to many? Utilitarianism is a trade-off between risks and benefits. Indeed, what kind of 'benefits' should we aim to maximise? And how do we measure a chosen benefit, and then balance its quantity versus quality? Applying utilitarianism may seem to support a wider use of lower-cost services but, with increasing medical advances, very expensive 'high-tech' procedures and 'wonder drugs' are becoming the norm in healthcare, consuming more resources to deliver the same utilitarian chosen benefits.

3. *Libertarian theory.*[8] This champions the principles of liberalism, autonomy, free choice and personal responsibility, in that individuals receive health benefits related to their contributions. In such a private, free-market system the government is less responsible for the distribution of the healthcare resources, and there are fewer public safety nets for the underprivileged. The US is one example, whereas many countries like Australia have both a public and a private healthcare system that balances healthcare needs.

4. *Prioritisation or favouring the worst-off theory.* The *sickest-first principle* is perhaps applicable to organ allocation and emergency department attention. It however, ignores posttreatment prognosis, and applies even when high costs are needed to achieve only minor gains. Some interventions (e.g. liver transplants) can be less effective for the sickest patients. The *youngest-first principle* has applications in organ transplantation

and kidney dialysis, but ignores prognosis. Also, should you prioritise an infant over an adolescent or a young adult, or indeed even over a productive middle-aged taxpayer?

5. *Social usefulness theory.*[9] The *instrumental value principle* prioritises individuals who promote important community values, but is open to abuse and is a social rather than ethical value. The *reciprocity principle* rewards usefulness or past sacrifice (e.g. living organ donors) but is irrelevant to acute care. Receiving priority care is perhaps relevant to healthcare staff who become sick from work; an example is the staff at Hong Kong's Prince of Wales Hospital who cared for contagious patients in the 2003 SARS epidemic.[10]

*

'That's all well and good, but these principles to choose who gets treated with what are subjective. How can that be fair?', Mike said.

I raised my beer can to acknowledge his point. 'I agree with you to a point. But doctors use their skills and expertise to assess, and they are generally reliable. There are also models, frameworks and guidelines to help.'

*

Models and guidelines for distributive justice

The theories and principles for equitable distribution have been applied in scoring systems to help allocate healthcare resources.

The *UNOS points* system is used by the non-profit organisation United Network for Organ Sharing, which coordinates US organ transplant activities. It is used for organ allocation, combining three principles: sickest-first, first-come, first-served (waiting time) and prognosis, but it is not directly relevant to resource considerations in acute medicine.

The *quality-adjusted life-year (QALY)* system is a form of utilitarian assessment. It takes into account both the quantity and the quality of life generated by healthcare interventions. It is the arithmetic product of life expectancy and a quality-of-life score for the remaining years, using a quality-of-life instrument such as the EQ-5D.[b] This is a simple questionnaire that a patient completes, with five questions on mobility, self-care, pain, usual activities and psychological status and with three possible answers for each item (1 = no problem, 2 = moderate problem, 3 = severe problem). A QALY places a time and quality-of-life measure in different health states. Comparisons can be made between interventions in disease groups, and priorities can be based on those interventions in a disease group that have better outcomes (higher QALYs) and are relatively inexpensive (low cost per QALY). Research in the use of QALYs for assessing allocation of acute care resources is continuing, but QALYs are as yet not useful for individual patient care.

The *disability-adjusted life-year (DALY)* system is a measure of disease burden from ill-health, expressed as the total number of years lost due to disability (YLD) plus years of life lost from early death (YLL). It is a way of measuring the population impact of a health problem, but has little relevance to individual acutely ill patients.

Distributive justice in clinical practice

In real life, at the individual patient level, doctors do not crank up apps on their computers or smart devices to calculate QALYs and DALYs. They do not have the time to calculate cost-effectiveness for every patient in need of care. Mike was right. Their decisions in allocating limited resources among patients are largely subjective, but clinical guidelines do exist to guide them (Chapter 5 Prognostications).

The American Medical Association counsels doctors to safeguard the welfare of their patients by supporting policies that allocate scarce healthcare resources fairly. They developed a Code of medical ethics opinion (11.1.3) – *Allocating limited health care resources*[12] – with the following criteria.

---

[b] Scores for the EQ-5D are generated from the ability of the individual to function in five dimensions: mobility, self-care, pain / discomfort, usual activities (work, study, housework, leisure activities), anxiety / depression, making a total of 243 possible health states, to which 'unconscious' and 'dead' are added to make 245 in total. The EQ-5D also includes self-marking a visual analogue scale on health status.[11]

(a) Base allocation policies on criteria relating to medical need, including urgency of need, likelihood and anticipated duration of benefit, and change in quality of life. In limited circumstances, it may be appropriate to take into consideration the amount of resources required for successful treatment. It is not appropriate to base allocation policies on social worth, perceived obstacles to treatment, patient contribution to illness, past use of resources, or other non-medical characteristics.

(b) Give first priority to those patients for whom treatment will avoid premature death or extremely poor outcomes, then to patients who will experience the greatest change in quality of life, when there are very substantial differences among patients who need access to the scarce resource(s).

(c) Use an objective, flexible, transparent mechanism to determine which patients will receive the resource(s) when there are not substantial differences among patients who need access to the scarce resource(s).

(d) Explain the applicable allocation policies or procedures to patients who are denied access to the scarce resource(s) and to the public.[12]

The processes by which healthcare decisions are made must be transparent, and the reasons for the decisions explicit. The exclusion of non-medical criteria in the decision making is universally followed. The UK Clinical Ethics Network states that differences in race, sex or income are not morally relevant to justify different treatment differences.[13] The National Health and Medical Research Council of Australia (NHMRC) recommends that all patients have equal access to basic health resources (with the right to choose private health resources). A just and equitable policy 'must also be sensitive to the needs of minority and marginalised groups' and should consider efficiency so as not to waste scarce resources.[14]

*

'We're chock-full!' our charge nurse Rosemary Smith said calmly but her furrowed forehead betrayed her anxiety. Thomas Wesley, Paul Constable and I had just finished our morning ward round and were enjoying coffee in the staff room.

'But we've just discharged two patients, Mrs Brown and Mr Aloysius', I replied.

'I know', Rosemary said, her eyes widened. 'We have four pending admissions. There is a young man in emergency with a ruptured spleen and fractured ribs from a motorbike accident. He's intubated, en route to surgery and will need to be admitted, and there are three elective-surgery booked admissions.' She rifled through the sheaf of papers she was holding. 'Here are the scheduled theatre lists today. Remember too that we're already two down on nurses; Jacinta's on maternity leave and Jo is sick.'

We huddled round to scrutinise the papers she produced. One booked admission was the neurosurgeons' removal of a large meningioma tumour. The second was the cardiac surgeons' repair of a heart valve. Both were urgent cases that needed postoperative ICU care.

'Tell theatre and Dr Benson's team that we cannot admit his gastric sleeve patient', I said to Rosemary. This was a 40-year-old man with morbid obesity, scheduled for bariatric stomach reduction surgery. Dr Benson would have to reschedule this non-urgent case, as the risks of postoperative complications would be increased without ICU care. 'We still need one more bed. Let's discharge the asthmatic young bloke in bed 11 back to a medical ward', I concluded. All the patients considered in our bed lottery ticked the criteria of achieving an improved quality of life and with a long-term benefit, but Dr Benson's patient lost on urgency of need.

Paul pursed his lips and shook his head. 'It's that dickhead Flintstone! All thanks to him', he said, echoing our thoughts. Dr David Flintstone (or 'Fred' by everyone else in the hospital) was the hospital's new CEO.

*

Each of the Australian states and territories determines allocations to its various health services, programs and medical research. By far, hospitals are the fat kids on the block, taking up the biggest piece of the cake. Each hospital's CEO and bean counters then allocate funding to respective departments. This is often and simply on a 'historical basis' where, in a good year, the ending year's budget is increased by the inflation rate, with prudent or profligate spending by departments usually being pragmatically overlooked. In a bad year, the increase, if any, is laughable. Replacement of equipment, or new equipment and additional services, is funded from a separate budget, determined by negotiations between department heads and the hospital administration. Prioritising such wide-ranging requests from such different disciplines makes the proverbial comparing 'apples with oranges' seem like, well, a piece of cake. In making their bids, department heads argue, cajole and plead, when guile and a strong personality are useful attributes. Of course, funding cuts impact adversely on patient care in one way or another, despite denials to the contrary by health bureaucrats. In the ICU this often affects bed capacity – that is, the number of patients who receive intensive care at any given time. If I were Mike's nana's ICU doctor, I could not prolong expensive futile treatment that would only delay death, and take up one ICU bed.

One of the worst fears of an ICU consultant is that of a 'full house', with no ICU beds available for the next critically ill patient. In every ICU, bed capacity is stretched by episodic peak demands, such as by severe influenza admissions in the winter months. Bed capacity is a resource, and managing optimal bed utilisation is a necessary aptitude for ICU doctors and nurses. Often, admissions become limited, and some incumbent patients are discharged to make way for new ones who are in more need of ICU care: a form of medical 'musical-beds'. Goals of care are thus changed that may impact on outcome. Some clinicians have examined the *queueing theory* – a mathematical study of problems that involve queuing for a service – to improve ICU bed access. Common strategies to do this are to reserve a 'last bed' for the utmost urgent emergency admission, decanting less-sick patients to 'spillover' beds in a high-dependency annex of the ICU (if indeed such beds are available), reserving a fixed number of beds for elective surgery admissions or cancelling elective surgery, as with Dr Benson's patient. None are ideal, always feasible or always practical; there are times when the ICU staff members need to make hard decisions.

Another factor that impacts on bed capacity is the availability of highly skilled ICU nurses. Nurse shortages can occur frequently that will contribute to reduced bed capacity. The new hospital CEO, Dr Flintstone, in his short reign of six months, had shown himself to be a control freak extraordinaire. To micromanage the hospital, he had doubled his administration staff, using a new '*Quality Assurance Funding Initiative*', which, when stripped of jargon, was simply a policy to transfer funds from clinical departments to his beloved Office of Executive Administration. This 'funding initiative' (or 'fucking initiative' as called by clinicians) stopped the engagement of private agency nurses as locums for those nurses on any leave, thus effectively cutting the ICU nurse numbers by four, and bed numbers by two.

Care in our healthcare system is modelled on the principles, categories and models of distributive justice. How we are treated may depend on the resources allocated to the hospital that we are admitted to. How big the health cake as decided by governments, how many portions as decided by state or territorial jurisdictions, how skinny a portion is sliced as decided by hospitals and, at the ground level, how the thin slices are consumed by departments and individual doctors will influence how we fare when we are sick, and how we may die.

*

Reflections

- Treating critical illness is expensive.
- Costs will influence hospital care and end-of-life care.
- Question: to whom should priority care be directed? Should this be those patients associated with the sickest status, the most urgent need, the best possible outcome, the most cost-effective care, the longest resulting life, the best quality of life attained, the next place in the queue, the youngest age, the oldest age or non-medical criteria (race, sex, income, social worth and past contributions)?
- Answer: all of the above, except for the last category. It's how the doctors decide.

References

1. Australian Institute of Health and Welfare. *Health expenditure Australia 2017–18*. Health and welfare expenditure series no. 65. Canberra, ACT: AIHW; 2019 https://aihw.gov.au.
2. World Health Organization. *Health expenditure country profiles 2017. Global health expenditure database*. Geneva: WHO; 2020. www.apps.who.int. › nha › database.
3. Independent Hospital Pricing Authority. *National hospital cost data collection cost report: round 22 financial year 2017–18*. Canberra, ACT: IHPA; 2020. https://ihpa.gov.au/sites/default/files/round_22_nhcdc_report_public_sector_round_22_2017-18_-_pdf_version.pdf.

4. Huynh TN, Kleerup EC, Wiley JF, Savitsky TD, Guse D, Garber BJ, et al. The frequency and cost of treatment perceived to be futile in critical care. *JAMA Intern Med* 2013;173(20):1887–94.

5. Bagshaw SM, Webb SA, Delaney A, George C, Pilcher D, Hart GK, et al. Very old patients admitted to intensive care in Australia and New Zealand: a multi-centre cohort analysis. *Crit Care* 2009;13(2):R45.

6. [No authors listed]. A controlled trial to improve care for seriously ill hospitalized patients. The study to understand prognoses and preferences for outcomes and risks of treatments (SUPPORT). *JAMA* 1995;274:1591–8.

7. Aristotle. *Politics*. Indianapolis: Hackett; 1998.

8. Olver IN. Limited resources limiting life? In: Olver IN, editor. *Is death ever preferable to life?* International Library of Ethics, Law, and the New Medicine. Dordrecht, Germany: Springer; 2002. pp. 120–42.

9. Persad G, Wertheimer A, Emanuel EJ. Principles for allocation of scarce medical interventions. *Lancet* 2009;373(9661):423–31.

10. Tomlinson B, Cockram C. SARS: experience at Prince of Wales Hospital, Hong Kong. *Lancet* 2003;361:1486–7.

11. National Institute for Health and Clinical Excellence. *Measuring effectiveness and cost effectiveness: the QALY*. London, UK: NICE; 2012.

12. American Medical Association. *Code of medical ethics. Opinion 11.1.3 – allocation of limited medical resources*. Chicago, IL: AMA; 2020.

13. UK Clinical Ethics Network. *Determining morally relevant reasons for treating people differently. Ethical issues – confidentiality/resource allocation/ethical considerations/maximising welfare/benefit*. 2011; 7 April. http://ukcen.net/ethical_issues/resource_allocation/ethical_considerations3.

14. National Health and Medical Research Council. *Ethical considerations relating to health care resource allocation decisions*. Canberra: NHMRC; 1993.

17

Medical mishaps

Deadly mistakes

Primum non nocere – above all, do no harm!

An axiom in the Hippocratic Oath by Hippocrates, but the
precise Latin and English expressions are attributed to Thomas
Sydenham (1624–89), an English physician

*

A medical mishap is a preventable adverse effect of care,
occurring particularly in hospitals. It may be a medical error due
to an individual's mistake, or it may be an unexpected accident
arising from a failing in the healthcare system (including equipment, resources and policies). The types and causes of mishaps
vary. They may not be evident, as 'near misses', or they may harm
the patient and contribute to or cause death. Fragile patients are
particularly vulnerable to medical mishaps. Hence consideration
of medical mishaps is relevant when reflecting on end-of-life
care.

*

Reports of incidents have been used to learn about medical
mishaps to improve patient safety. Incident reporting systems,
however, are based on voluntary reporting in a non-punitive

environment, and may reveal only a percentage of errors. Other methods to capture errors include reviews by peers in department meetings or of patient medical records, patient interviews and analyses of insurance malpractice claims. Despite an introduction by the World Health Organization of a standardised set of patient safety concepts – the International Classification of Patient Safety, ICPS[1] – there is inconsistency between countries in collecting and comparing data on medical mishaps. One reason is the diversity of terms used to label medical errors. Jurisdictions use the terms below.

Terminology

- *Adverse event* – is the most commonly used term for medical mishaps, defined as 'an unintended injury resulting in prolonged hospitalisation, disability or death caused by healthcare delivery'. Subcategories include *preventable*, *ameliorable* (could have been less harmful if care had been different), *near-miss* or *potential adverse* event (averted by early detection or luck) and causative *acts of commission* or *omission*.
- *Critical (or clinical) incident* – is similar to an adverse event but also includes 'near-miss' events and hazards in the healthcare environment that expose patients to harm.
- *Sentinel event* – is a major adverse event: a clinical incident that directly caused, or could have caused, death or serious injury, unrelated to any pre-existing condition or risk inherent in the treatment. Australia recognises eight core sentinel events (*see Box 1*).

1. Sentinel Events – Australia
1. Procedures involving the wrong patient or body part.
2. Suicide of a patient.
3. Retained instruments or material after surgery requiring reopening.
4. Intravascular gas embolism.
5. Blood transfusion incompatibility with haemolytic reaction.
6. Medication error causing death.
7. Maternal death in pregnancy and birth.
8. Infant discharged to wrong family.

- *Unplanned re-admission* – to the same hospital within 28 days following a surgical procedure, due to unexpected complications attributable to the procedure, e.g. bleeding, infection and malfunction of implants.
- *Hospital-acquired diagnoses*[2] – identify numbers and types of complications by diagnostic codes without relying on voluntary reports. Hospital medical records routinely code patients' diagnoses according to the *International Classification of Diseases* (ICD-10-AM). The *Classification of Hospital Acquired Diagnoses* (CHADx) further classifies ICD-10-AM codes into a hierarchy of 17 classes (with subclasses) of adverse-event diagnoses. Hospital coders review medical records to flag adverse events that occur (i.e. are 'acquired') in hospital, and this flagged CHADx code designates the class of hospital-acquired diagnosis.

Incidence

Due to variations in terminology, definitions and measurement of adverse events across countries and jurisdictions, clear and consistent data on incidences of medical mishaps are difficult to pinpoint. In the US, the Institute of Medicine published a landmark report in 1999 that up to 98,000 patients die each year because of mistakes in hospitals, based on 1984 data.[3] In 2010, the US Office of Inspector General for Health and Human Services said that bad hospital care contributed to the deaths of 180,000 patients in Medicare each year.[4] A controversial US study in 2013 looked at studies from 2008 to 2011 and reported that 210,000 deaths per year were associated with preventable harm in hospitals, with an estimated true number of over 440,000 per year.[5] That estimate would make medical mishaps the third leading cause of death in America, behind heart disease and cancer. In 2000 the UK Chief Medical Officer reported that 850,000 adverse events occurred in the NHS (National Health Service) each year.[6] Although death figures were not given, deaths of over 40,000 each year could be extrapolated. A 2018 UK study reported that 237 million medication errors occur in the NHS each year, with avoidable adverse drug reactions contributing to between 1700 and 22,303 deaths.[7] Large international reviews of patient charts in multiple countries (the US, UK, Canada, Australia, New Zealand, Spain, Sweden and the Netherlands)[8] estimate that between 4% and

17% of hospital admissions are associated with an adverse event, with one- to two-thirds being preventable. From the majority of reports, the median incidence of adverse events in hospitals globally is approximately 10%, of which 14% of events result in permanent disability and 7% in death.[9] Almost half are said to be preventable.

In Australia, the government's Productivity Commission 2018 report[10] showed a total of 10.6 million hospital admissions for 2015–16, of which 6.6% of public hospital separations and 3.8% of private hospital separations reported adverse events; data of the two groups are not comparable because of different casemixes and recording practices. The most common adverse event groups reported for public hospital separations were procedures (50%) and adverse effects of medications (38%). Surgical care had higher rates of adverse events than other types of care (7.7% and 4.7% respectively). Nationwide, there were 82 sentinel events resulting in death or very serious harm, a 'reasonably comforting' very low incidence of 7.7 per million hospital separations.[10]

Common adverse events and causes

The common adverse events are shown in *Box 2*.

2. Common Adverse Events
• Mishaps to patients during surgical and medical care
• Infection following a procedure
• Haemorrhage and haematoma complicating a procedure
• Other diagnoses of complications of medical and surgical care
• Selected postprocedural disorders
• Complications of implants and prosthetic devices
• Adverse effects of medications (misuse, anaphylaxis)
• Blood and blood products transfusion reactions
• Procedures causing abnormal reactions/complications
• Falls
• Pressure ulcers

In reviewing adverse events, causes can be considered under a framework of causal contributing factors (*see Box 3*). There may be overlap, such as a mix of staff error, poor supervision and equipment failure. Human behavioural failure is the most common cause, but should not be the only point of attention. Conditions in the healthcare system often enable the adverse event, and reviews to prevent future recurrences must also consider latent (organisational) factors to improve training, policies and procedures.

| 3. Adverse Events – Framework of Causal and Contributing Factors ||
Causal	Contributing factors
Individual staff members	Knowledge, skills, motivation, cognition, communication, experience, stress, fatigue
Organisational	Staffing level, supervision, resources, ward environment, policies, safety culture, workload, administrative support, equipment availability and malfunction
Patient-related	Condition, co-morbidity, age, mobility, language, distress, culture, communication, length of stay

Root cause analysis

Reporting of adverse events are mandatory in all jurisdictions, and they require investigation, including root cause analysis (RCA) reviews. This is a method that looks for the 'root of the problem' in the health system failure. A number of factors can usually be identified as causes of the adverse event. The root cause is one which, if eliminated, prevents the adverse event from recurring. If eliminating a factor benefits, but does not prevent, the adverse event from recurring, it is causal and not a root cause. RCA is a structured process to answer what happened, why it happened and what actions will prevent or minimise a recurrence of the root cause. One technique is the '*five whys*', which asks at least five questions why a causal factor presented. Each question addresses the answer to the previous question. In this way, successive layers of causal factors are peeled back to arrive at a bottom root cause. The '*fishbone*' is another RCA technique, credited to Dr Ishikawa, a Japanese quality control expert. The adverse event is the fish head and possible causes are skeletal bones attached

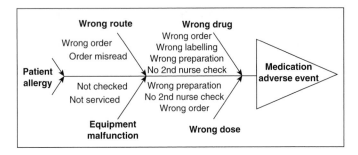

Fig. 17.1   A fishbone RCA of a medication adverse event.

to the spine. Each cause, plus factors giving rise, to the cause is ranked, and then examined and excluded to derive the root cause. Fig. 17.1 is an example of a fishbone RCA of a medication adverse event.

*

The monthly peer review meeting of the departments of intensive care, anaesthesia and surgery specialties presented a case each from plastic surgery and general surgery. A 70-year-old man presented for surgery on his right fourth finger to correct its contracture due to Dupytren disease – an abnormal thickening and tightening of the fascia beneath the skin of the palm and fingers. The plastic surgeon completed the procedure successfully on the patient's right *middle* finger that also had an early contracture. The patient had not requested or consented to surgery on that middle digit. During the Universal Protocol timeout, the presurgery verification process in theatre, the surgeon's assistant had used a marking pen to mark the site of surgery as per protocol. She wrote 'Y' on the patient's right palm instead of on the right fourth finger. The surgeon thought that he had to operate on the middle finger and nobody questioned his decision. This was an adverse event, albeit not disastrous, as surgery was scheduled a month later for the right fourth finger.

The second case was a 50-year-old female who presented for cholecystectomy (or removal of the gall bladder). In the past month, she had experienced severe abdominal pains with indigestion, nausea and vomiting. Her GP diagnosed cholecystitis, or inflammation of the gall bladder, and referred her for its removal (cholecystectomy). The general surgeon operated by laparoscopy ('keyhole' surgery) and could not find a gall bladder; it had been previously removed. The patient, a recent immigrant from Asia, spoke little English. Her daughter had acted as a translator in communicating with doctors and nurses, but no one had asked her whether her mother had undergone previous gall bladder surgery. Her mother suffered an unnecessary procedure, but fortunately no untoward injury. Both cases demonstrated the 'Swiss cheese' effect of multiple small errors to cause an adverse event (see next section). The red faces at the peer review meeting did not, and could not, offer any excuse.

*

Swiss cheese errors

Why do adverse events still happen today when hospitals have evolved safety strategies over the past 30 years, honed by lessons from past events? The reason is, if a key step in the process fails, it may not be mitigated by other parts of the system. A deviation from procedure may then be unrecoverable, and a mishap occurs despite layers of safeguards. James Reason, a professor of psychology at the University of Manchester, UK, proposed a 'Swiss cheese' analogy of how mishaps occur in latent conditions.[11] In a complex system, hazards are prevented from occurring by a series of barriers. Each barrier has unintended weaknesses or 'holes', as depicted by layered slices of Swiss cheese. These weaknesses are unpredictable, with holes opening and closing at random. When, by chance, all slices of cheese become aligned through one hole in each and every slice, the safety barriers are breached and the mishap occurs to cause the patient harm. The focus is the healthcare system rather than the individual, and the model captures random causal factors as well as deliberate acts.

A key point of the Swiss cheese model is that, by preventing any one hole to line up, the eventual adverse event could have been prevented. These holes include aspects of skill sets, workload, workflow, training, equipment and communication. The two cases presented at the peer review meeting above are examples. Multiple checks of patient identification and surgical procedure are designed to prevent wrong site surgery and wrong procedures. The first check is conducted when the patient arrives at the operating theatre suite reception. Then, when ready, the patient is wheeled into the operating theatre, where the 'holy trinity' – nurse, anaesthetist and surgeon – conduct a second check called 'timeout'. This includes the surgeon marking the precise site of surgery, and not just the correct limb, as was done in the first case. Similarly in the second case of a missing gall bladder, no one had asked the patient about prior surgery; a 'hole alignment' from the GP to the operating table! Administering blood transfusions is another example of potential Swiss cheese mishaps; holes include incorrect labelling, wrong blood bag delivered and incomplete patient checks by two staff members. The Swiss cheese model is also used in industry, such as airlines and pilots, to promote a culture of safety.

Human and financial costs

Adverse events exact a high human as well as financial toll. Consequent additional hospital stays cost the UK NHS £2000 million a year, and litigation claims an extra £400 million in 2002; the extra cost to health services in the US was from US$17,000 million to US$29,000 million annually.[12] The cost of harm (flow-on and indirect) includes loss of productivity, and for the US in 2008 was estimated to be almost US$1 trillion.[13] In the Australian State of Victoria, adverse events in 2003–04 (6.9% of hospital admissions) reportedly added A$6826 to the cost of each admission, totalling A$460,311 million or 15.7% of the total expenditure on direct hospital costs,[14] a figure generally applicable globally.[13] Patient harm is the 14th leading cause of the global disease burden, comparable to chronic conditions like some cancers.[13] Many adverse events are preventable, and the costs of prevention are miniscule in comparison to adverse consequences. Improving patient safety in US Medicare hospitals is estimated to have saved US$28 billion between 2010 and 2015.[13]

A systems approach to mishaps

The push for safe and quality healthcare began in the 1970s. Today, patients in hospitals should consequently be safer from medical errors, but are they? Data across jurisdictions are inconsistent, varied and hard to compare, but there is no dependable hard evidence to show that safety has progressed significantly – for example, in terms of reduced percentage of adverse events (although this may be explained by more reportings of incidents). Strategies in minimising mishaps have previously concentrated on human errors, with voluntary reporting and reviewing of errors the mainstay methods. This addresses deficiencies in skill sets and is an individualistic approach. However, most adverse events, particularly adverse drug events, are attributable to system failures and are not the result of negligence or poor training alone.[12] Today, conceptual thinking on healthcare safety takes a systems approach focusing on deficiencies in the healthcare system – that is, in design, organisation, operation and culture – rather than on individual providers or individual services.[15] Simply striving for personnel to be perfect, or punishing individuals who make mistakes, will not appreciably improve patient safety. This systems approach places emphasis on every component of patient safety to offer the most effective range of risk reduction solutions and, in doing so, improves the healthcare system itself and constructs nationwide programs. Reviews use methods of data capture that do not rely on voluntary reporting of adverse events, such as patient reviews and hospital-acquired diagnoses (see earlier section). Nonetheless, voluntary reporting of adverse events remains vital and, with it, confidentiality of accounts. While necessary to promote incident reporting and to protect patients and staff involved, data on performance between groups or hospitals have to remain inaccessible to the public, and even to individual doctors. To the consumer, choosing doctors and hospitals (if applicable) is not made easier.

*

'She's written another article,' my wife said, handing over to me the latest issue of the paper 'Community news'. Di was referring to the front-page piece by Joan Blade, the doctor-unfriendly health journalist. The headline screamed, '*Another doctor bungle*'.

*

> **Reflections**
>
> - Adverse events in hospital are still too common, at around 10 incidents per 100 admissions (global median). Some are sentinel events resulting in serious disability or death. Up to half are reported to be preventable
> - There is no universal standardisation of terms and definitions across countries.
> - The personal and financial costs of adverse events are massive, and the costs of harm dwarf those of preventive measures.
> - Strategies to improve safety in healthcare should include voluntary and non-voluntary recording of incidents, using a systems approach to review deficiencies in the whole healthcare system, rather than looking only at the performance of individuals.

References

1. World Health Organization. *The conceptual framework for the International Classification for Patient Safety (ICPS)*. Geneva: WHO; 2010.
2. Utz M, Johnston T, Halech R. *A review of the Classification of Hospital Acquired Diagnoses (CHADx)*. Brisbane, QLD: Health Statistic Unit, Queensland Health; 2012.
3. Institute of Medicine (US) Committee on Quality of Health Care in America, Kohn LT, Corrigan JM, Molla S, Donaldson MS, editors. *To err is human: building a safer health system*. Washington, DC: National Academy Press; 1999.
4. Office of Inspector General. *Adverse events in hospitals: national incidence among Medicare beneficiaries*. Washington, DC: Department of Health and Human Services; 2010.
5. James JT. A new, evidence-based estimate of patient harms associated with hospital care. *J Patient Saf* 2013;9(3):122–8.
6. Department of Health. *An organisation with a memory*. Report of an expert group on learning from adverse events in the NHS chaired by the Chief Medical Officer. London, UK: DOH; 2000.
7. Elliot R, Camacho E, Campbell F, Jankovic D, St James M, et al; Policy Research Unit in Economic Evaluation of Health and Care Interventions; EEPRU. *Prevalence and economic burden of medication errors in the NHS in England*. Sheffield and York, Yorks, UK: Universities of Sheffield and York; 2018.
8. Rafter N, Hickey A, Condell S, Conroy R, O'Connor P, Vaughan D, et al. Adverse events in healthcare: learning from mistakes. *Q J Med* 2015;108(4):273–7.

9. de Vries EN, Ramrattan MA, Smorenburg SM, Gouma DJ, Boermeester MA. The incidence and nature of in-hospital adverse events: a systematic review. *Qual Saf Health Care* 2008;17(3):216–23.

10. Productivity Commission. *Report on government services 2018*. Health. Part E. Canberra: Australian Government; 30 January 2018.

11. Reason J. Human error: models and management. *BMJ* 2000; 320(7237):768–70.

12. World Health Assembly. *Quality of care: patient safety*. Report by the Secretariat. Geneva: WHO, March 2002.

13. Slawomirski L, Auraaen A, Klazinga N. *The economics of patient safety*. Paris: OECD; 2017. http://www.oecd.org/els/health-systems/The-economics-of-patient-safety-March-2017.pdf.

14. Ehsani JP, Jackson T, Duckett SJ. The incidence and cost of adverse events in Victorian Hospitals 2003–04. *Med J Aust* 2006;184(11):551–5.

15. Agency for Healthcare Research and Quality, Patient Safety Network. *Patient safety 101/the systems approach to analyzing patient safety*. Rockville, MD: AHRQ, US Department of Health and Human Services; 2019. https://psnet.ahrq.gov.

Glossary and Acronyms

ACD advance care directive or advance directive – living will
ACSQHC Australian Commission on Safety and Quality in Health Care
A&E accident and emergency (UK)
ALS amyotrophic lateral sclerosis; a form of motor neuron disease
ANZICS Australian and New Zealand Intensive Care Society
APACHE II Acute Physiologic and Chronic Health Evaluation II
ARDS adult respiratory distress syndrome
Ca carcinoma or cancer
CHADx Classification of Hospital Acquired Diagnoses
CICM College of Intensive Care Medicine
COPD chronic obstructive pulmonary disease
CPR cardiopulmonary resuscitation
CT computed tomography
CVP central venous pressure
DALY disability-adjusted life-year
DBD (organ) donation by brain death
DCD (organ) donation by circulatory or cardiac death
DNAR do not attempt resuscitation
DNR do not resuscitate
DPMP donors per million population
ED emergency department UK
EEG electroencephalogram
ENT ear, nose and throat
ER emergency room (US)
EVAR endovascular aneurysm repair
GMC General Medical Council
GP general practitioner
grey zone a term for the terminal phase of life
HDU high-dependency unit
ICD International Classification of Diseases (ICD-10-AM)
ICPS International Classification of Patient Safety
ICU intensive care unit
IFA Islamic Fiqh Academy
IV intravenous

MCS minimally conscious state
MMR measles, mumps and rubella
MPM Mortality Probability Model
NFR not for resuscitation
NHMRC National Health and Medical Research Council
NHS National Health Service (UK)
OIC Organization of the Islamic Conference
OTA Organ and Tissue Authority
PCO_2 carbon dioxide tension in blood; denotes degree of spontaneous breathing and carbon dioxide retention.
PO_2 oxygen tension in blood; denotes oxygenation level
PTSD posttraumatic stress disorder
PVS persistent vegetative state
QALY quality-adjusted life-year
RCA root cause analysis
RMO resident medical officer
SAPS Simplified Acute Physiology Score
SDM substitute decision maker
Trachy tracheostomy
twilight zone a term for the terminal phase of life
ventilator respirator
YLD years lost due to disability
YLL years of life lost from early death

Index

Page numbers followed by "*f*" indicate figures, "*t*" indicate tables, and "*b*" indicate boxes.

216